DARK ANGELS

Robert Dando

Published by
Chipmunkapublishing
PO Box 6872
Brentwood
Essex CM13 1ZT
United Kingdom

http://www.chipmunkapublishing.com

PART ONE

DARK ANGELS

Chapter ONE

Brenda got out of the cab, and paid off the driver. The cab drove off into the night. Slowly and unsteadily, Brenda walked up the front steps of the police station, and made her way inside.

Luckily, there was no one else at the reception counter who was waiting to be attended to. Brenda walked up to the uniformed police officer behind the counter.

“Yes, can I help you?” he asked.

Suddenly, everything seemed to be swimming in front of Brenda’s eyes.

“Yes, I’d like to speak to someone about...” she began.

But that was as far as she managed to get before she fainted.

****

Slowly, she came back to consciousness.

When she had finally come too, she found herself seated in a chair beside a table in an interview room. A man was hovering close beside her.

“Are you feeling all right now?” he asked, anxiously. “Or would you like us to get you an ambulance to take you to hospital?”

"Oh no, that won't be necessary, thanks," she replied. "I'll be all right in a moment, it's just that I've been under a lot of strain, recently."

"I expect you could do with a hot drink, Ms…."

"Dalton. Brenda Dalton. Yes thanks, I'll have a cup of coffee."

"How do you take it? Black or white?"

"White, with two sugars, please."

When the coffee arrived, Brenda gratefully drank almost all of it in one gulp, seemingly oblivious to the fluid's hot temperature.

"Thanks, I really needed that" she said.

"Now, are you sure you don't want an ambulance? Are you sure you don't want to go to hospital?" the man persisted.

"No, really, I'm alright," said Brenda "I'm very tired, but I don't need to go to hospital. I came here because I wanted to talk to someone in authority, and I don't want to pass up that opportunity, now I'm here."

"Well, you can talk to me. I'm in authority here," said the man, smiling. "My name's Donaldson. Inspector Donaldson. Now, what was it you wanted to talk to me about?"

"Well, it's all rather a long story, really," said Brenda. "I am... well, I'm going to resign, but at the moment, strictly speaking, I still <u>am</u> a student nurse at that mental hospital, the one further up off the motorway. Do you know it?"

"Yes."

"Well, I told you it was a long story, Inspector," said Brenda, "and it is...."

Chapter TWO

I won't bore you, Inspector, with any of the reasons why I wanted to become a mental nurse in the first place. Anyway, the whole thing's rather academic now, because I'll never progress beyond the stage of being a student. As I told you just now, I'm going to resign. I haven't told <u>them</u> yet, but that's what I'm going to do. I'll phone them tomorrow and tell them I'm not going back there again, not ever. I never want to set foot in that hospital again. I'll post all my books and uniforms back to them. I know it'll cost a bit in postage and packing, but I don't care about that. Just so long as the place is out of my life for good, that's the main thing.

****

Almost immediately after I'd started working at the hospital – my very first day there, in fact – I could see that things weren't the way they should be, not ideally.

For a start, there didn't really seem to be any psychotherapy to speak of, or any talking treatments, either; basically, the nurses would just dish out drugs to the patients all the time. And I really believe those drugs were over-prescribed; the women patients became almost like zombies. (By the way, the hospital doesn't have any mixed sex wards, only female wards, where I worked, and male wards).

I suppose in a way it hardly mattered if the patients were almost like zombies, because there didn't really seem to be any set agenda or set programme of activities for them, anyway. Basically, they were just herded into the television lounge each day, and then they were seated in chairs, where most of them would then just stare into space all day long. Oh, it was true that the television, in the corner of the room, was on all day, but it was turned so low that you couldn't really hear anything that was being said on it, anyway. What a waste of good electricity, I thought. Either they should turn it up so everyone can hear it properly, or else they should turn it off and give all these patients something more constructive to do with their time...

I once tried to raise these points with one of the other nurses. But all she said was: "Why complain about it? It only means less work for us, the way we do these things now. Don't look a gift horse in the mouth."

Another thing that didn't seem right was the fact that the doctor hardly ever visited the ward. This meant, in effect, that everything was run by the nurses – in particular, Senior Nurse Rawsthorne...

I could tell at our first meeting that she didn't like me. And I didn't like her, either. But I didn't know just how unlikeable she could be – or rather, just how evil she could be – until I saw the way that she treated one of the patients. Her name's Dorothy Little...

****

Inspector, I don't know if you recall the Dorothy Little case? She killed her husband. She claimed she had done it out of self-defence, as a way of stopping his constant battering of her. Unfortunately, no one had ever seen him batter her; he had never admitted it to, or boasted about it to, anyone; and, just as bad, <u>she</u> had never complained about it to anyone, either. Not that there was necessarily anything suspicious about her not complaining; it's not exactly the easiest thing in the world for anyone to have to talk about. But it was really this previous silence on her part, unsuspicious though it may have been, which led to the jury not believing her. (If only more people realised how difficult it can be to talk about these things). She was convicted of murder. Because of the way she'd killed him – she stabbed him several times, and while he was asleep, moreover – there were doubts raised about her sanity. So instead of being sent to prison, she was ordered to be detained indefinitely, either at a secure mental hospital, or at least at a secure unit within a mental hospital.

Well at this point, she began to protest loudly that what she'd done, had been done in self-defence; that she hadn't committed murder either as a sane person <u>or</u> as an insane one; and that she wasn't insane, anyway. Then she seemed to lose control of herself and she started yelling abuse, first at the judge, and then at the jury, and then she carried on yelling as she was removed from the dock by the wardens in charge of her. All in all, perhaps it wasn't, on reflection, exactly the best way of trying to convince people that she wasn't really insane.

Of course, she could have been sent to Broadmoor, or one of the other top security mental hospitals that we've got in this country. But instead it was considered sufficient to send her to a local secure unit. Our hospital had a locked ward. And so, accordingly, she was sent there. I suppose many people would have said she was really very lucky in being sent to us, as opposed to being sent to one of the top security mental hospitals, considering the bad reputations that those places can sometimes have.

Well, maybe she would have been lucky – if only it hadn't been for Senior Nurse Rawsthorne…

****

It so happened that Dorothy Little was the only patient on the locked ward at the particular time that I was working at the hospital. Of course, there were other committed patients in the hospital, but they were all confused, elderly women who had been committed for their own safety, and not because they were considered to be dangerous to anyone else. It had been decided that it would be sufficient for them to be kept in the normal (now no jokes, Inspector, about that word, please) female psychogeriatric ward. By contrast, Dorothy was the only committed patient in the hospital who was considered to be dangerous to other people, and the only committed patient, moreover, who actively wanted to be released from the place.

I would later find out that there was one other important thing about her, namely that she never had any visitors. For a start, both of her parents were dead, and she had been an only child. And the few friends, that she had, turned out to be of the strictly fair weather sort; as soon as she was put in hospital, they just dropped her like a hot potato. Maybe they couldn't really be blamed. No one relishes being associated with a diagnosed loony. It was an association that might have proved to be detrimental in some way or other.

So anyway, there she was, desperate to get out of the hospital, but unable to do so; all alone in the world, with no one to speak up for her; no one to protest on her behalf about anything that was done to her. All in all, a perfect target for a bully like Senior Nurse Rawsthorne. As I would soon witness – quite memorably…

Just about everything that Dorothy did was supervised, even if it wasn't really necessary, Rawsthorne claimed it <u>was</u> necessary. And even when she wasn't doing the supervising herself, it was being done by one of those nurses who could be counted on as being among her cronies. I'm sure you'll agree, Inspector, that we all need privacy, at least some of the time. It's a bit much when you can's even go to the toilet without having a nurse hovering about outside the cubicle who can hear you relieving yourself.

But, as I would soon discover, bathtimes could be an even worse experience for Dorothy.

When I was assigned, on one occasion, to assist in supervising Dorothy during her bathtime, I thought that at most I would be one of only two nurses carrying out this duty. I wouldn't have thought that more than two nurses would have been necessary. But in fact, there were four of us: Rawsthorne, two of her cronies, and me. I'm not really sure why they included me. Maybe they wanted to discover if I would turn out to be just like them; maybe they wanted to find out whether I could be admitted into their inner circle, so to speak. Well, they would soon be disillusioned on that score.

"Right," said Rawsthorne to Dorothy. "Get undressed."

There were no screens behind which Dorothy could go; there was no kind of private area at all. We were all just standing around the bathtub. Slowly and reluctantly, Dorothy started to comply. It wasn't the easiest thing in the world to do, with Rawsthorne and the other nurses staring at her. It became even more difficult for her after she had stripped down to bra and knickers, but finally she managed to remove those garments as well.

Now, we've all had that nightmare, at some time, haven't we, Inspector? I mean the nightmare of being naked in a public place, when everyone else around you is fully clothed. It might not be so bad if your body is attractive. But Dorothy's wasn't.

Not that I would consider myself to be a particularly good judge of what it is that makes a woman's body attractive. Me, I'm strictly heterosexual, Inspector. I only know what I like to look for in men's bodies. But even I could tell that Dorothy wouldn't exactly have made it onto page three of the Sun.

To describe her from the top down; her arms were dumpy. Her breasts sagged, her stomach stuck out so much that she could only be described as being potbellied. She had very thick thighs. Her pubic hair was a tangled, sprawling mass of thick black curls. Her legs were dumpy, just like her arms. And she had varicose veins.

And just then, Rawsthorne and the other nurses started giggling at Dorothy.

A very nasty look came into her eyes. Her breathing got deeper, and she clenched her fists, obviously having to control herself with a great effort.

Now don't do anything silly, Dorothy, I thought. Don't let them provoke you...

"Don't be violent," said Rawsthorne, almost as an echo of my thoughts. "Don't even think about it. And don't leave your clothes all over the floor like that. Pick them up, fold them up and put them on that," she finished, indicating a chair in the corner of the room.

For a long moment, Dorothy looked at her silently, as if debating in her mind as to whether letting rip would be worth the inevitable retaliation. Then finally, evidently deciding that it wouldn't be worth it after all, she relaxed. She bent down to pick up her clothes.

And in doing so, she broke wind. Personally, I would have to say it was one of the loudest farts that I had ever heard; an absolute ripsnorter.

That tore it. Rawsthorne and the other nurses burst into screams of laughter. Dorothy screamed too, only her scream was one of rage, not laughter. She lunged at Rawsthorne, punching and kicking her.

Which was just the sort of excuse they all needed for what they did next.

They grabbed her by her arms and legs. I didn't join in. Rawsthorne shouted: "Get a straightjacket, Dalton! You know where they're kept!" But I couldn't move. I seemed to be rooted to the spot. Eventually one of the other nurses rushed off to get the garment in question, and then the three of them gradually managed to put it on the naked, struggling, woman in their grasp. Then they removed her to the seclusion room. Her arms may have been immobilised by then, but she was still capable of kicking and screaming. And she continued to do plenty of both. But they got her into the seclusion room and then left, shutting and bolting the door after them.

Rawsthorne glared at me.

"Where the hell were you while all that was going on"? she said.

****

As I said earlier, Inspector, I think the reason Rawsthorne included me, among the nurses supervising Dorothy, was because she wanted to find out whether I wanted to join in her little games. After what happened, it must have become very clear that I didn't. As a result, I suspect she decided, from then on, to confine her victimisation of Dorothy, and any other patients who provided her with the same sorts of opportunities, to those occasions when I wasn't present.

I think the reason I was present, the next time, was simply because it was a form of persecution which Rawsthorne hadn't planned in advance; instead, she simply took advantage of an opportunity that was suddenly presented to her.

It was a little while later. I heard Dorothy suddenly call out: "Nurse! Nurse!"

Rawsthorne and I happened to be in different rooms at the time. She heard Dorothy was well. Rawsthorne and I simultaneously approached the door of the seclusion room from different directions. The door had a sliding panel which could be opened and closed from the outside. (Obviously, not from the inside as well; otherwise, any unstraitjacketed patient could open it, reach out, and unbolt the door). Rawsthorne opened the panel and we both looked in. Dorothy was standing by the door, in her straightjacket, and naked from the waist downwards.

"What do you want?" said Rawsthorne.

"My nose is running," said Dorothy.

Indeed it was. Quite profusely, in fact. I expect it was the result of repeated sneezing. Indeed, when Dorothy opened her mouth to speak, some of the stuff from her nose got into her mouth, and she had to spit it out again. Much to Rawsthorne's amusement, I noticed.

The two nurses, who had been present in the bathroom, were loitering nearby with a third, an elderly little nurse named Evans. Rawsthorne beckoned them to come across to her. The two nurses, who had been in the bathroom, came over, though Evans remained where she was.

"Your nose is running? Then why don't you wipe it?" said Rawsthorne. "Oh, of course, I'm sorry. I forgot. You can't, can you?"

The other two nurses started giggling, just as they had in the bathroom.

I backed away. I didn't want to be part of this. I could see that Evans looked as disgusted as I felt.

Rawsthorne asked the two other nurses in turn whether they had a spare tissue, and again, in turn, each of them answered in the negative, in obviously mock-apologetic tones. (Rawsthorne didn't ask Evans or me, I noticed).

"I've got a tissue here," said Rawsthorne. She produced it, nice and clean, from the pocket of her uniform, and held it up so that Dorothy could see it. "I could come in and wipe your nose for you. Would you like me to do that?"

Dorothy didn't reply. I could only assume that her desire to ease her physical discomfort was battling against her reluctance to demean herself by having to grovel to that uniformed excuse for a human being.

"You heard me, didn't you?" said Rawsthorne. "I said, would you like that?"

"Yes," Dorothy muttered. Evidently, her desire to ease her discomfort had triumphed over her distaste for grovelling.

"I think you missed out a little word or two."

"Yes please."

"I think you mean: "Yes please, Ms Rawsthorne" Don't you?"

"Yes please, Ms Rawsthorne."

"Are you sorry you attacked me in the bathroom?"

"Yes, Ms. Rawsthorne."

"Then say it."

"I'm sorry I attacked you, Ms Rawsthorne."

"And you'll never do it again, will you?"

"No, Ms Rawsthorne."

"Promise?"

"I promise, Ms Rawsthorne."

"Good," said Rawsthorne. She paused for a moment, and then she went on: "Oh yes, I almost forgot, silly of me. The tissue. As I was saying, I could come in and wipe your nose for you. But I'm afraid I need the tissue for myself. I've only got the one." Whereupon she blew her own nose very loudly, and then said: "Ah, that's better! There's nothing worse that having a runny nose, is there?

I'll tell you what: why don't you just rub your nose on the wall? That should do the trick."

At this point, Dorothy started screaming obscenities at Rawsthorne. On and on they went, including threats to hill Rawsthorne…

I felt the bile start to rise in my throat. I clapped my hand over my mouth, and I ran off to the lavatory, as fast as I could. I heard Rawsthorne saying: "It looks like Dalton just can't take it." This provoked laughter from the other two nurses.

I only just managed to get to the toilet bowl in time before I threw up.

Chapter THREE

I don't think it's any exaggeration to say, Inspector, that I had never been so sick in all my life as I was, on that particular occasion. (Though as things turned out, there would be a later occasion when I would feel even sicker. But I don't want to run ahead of myself. I'll be coming to that in due course).

After I had managed to get my bearings again, I flushed the toilet, and then I sat down on it. Not because I needed to use it, but simply because I needed to sit down. I felt as if my legs would otherwise give way underneath me.

For Christ's sake, just what sort of place *was* this hospital, I thought to myself? And just what sort of monster was that Rawsthorne woman? What stone had *she* crawled out from under? She couldn't be a human being, surely!

After I had recovered somewhat, I slowly got to my feet, and I *mean* slowly. I wasn't quite sure if I was capable yet of standing on my own two feet without collapsing to the floor. But fortunately I was. I took a deep breath. Then I slowly walked to the door, opened it, and peeped out.

Just for a moment, I wondered if it had all been some horrible nightmare of some kind. The corridor, you see, was completely deserted, and everything seemed to be silent. It was as if none of it had really happened.

But the very next moment, I knew it definitely hadn't been a dream.

As I said, the corridor was deserted.

But things were <u>not</u> silent. Not totally.

I could hear the quiet sound of sobbing coming from the seclusion room.

I crossed to the door, I slid open the panel, and I looked in. Dorothy was crouched in the corner of the room, weeping. Even from where I was standing, I could make out certain marks on the wall, which suggested to me that she had actually been reduced to trying to put Rawsthorne's suggestion into effect, in an effort to clean her nose. But it didn't really seem to have done her any good. If anything, things had become worse; if anything her nasal substances were spread out over her face, even more than they had been before.

Now, of course, I knew that I didn't have the authority to go in that room and take the straitjacket off her. I was only a student, after all. But I didn't see why I couldn't at least go in there and clean up her face for her. I knew there was a risk that Rawsthorne might come along and catch me at it; and that if she did, she would be bound to give me hell. But just then, I didn't really care about that. At that precise moment in time, I was too angry to care about that; or indeed to care about anything, other than trying to bring some comfort to that poor woman sobbing in the corner of that room.

After I had taken a quick look round, to make sure no one could see me, I unbolted the door, and I walked in.

Dorothy looked up, and her expression of misery was instantly replaced by one of alarm, if not one of terror.

"Don't hurt me," she whimpered. "I beg of you, please don't hurt me..."

Clearly, by this time, she was afraid of anyone who was wearing a nurse's uniform.

I felt really angry inside. For Christ's sake, what kind of hospital was it that could reduce someone to this sort of state, I thought to myself? Surely this didn't come under the heading of cure or therapy, did it?

"It's all right, Dorothy," I said. "I'm a friend." I produced a packet of tissues from my pocket. Luckily, I had only had to use one or two of them since I'd originally opened the packet, which meant that most of them were still available to be used. "Do you see these? I've got some tissues here, just for you. Nice, clean tissues. Now come on, let's get your face cleaned up." So saying, I proceeded to wipe her face as well as I could with the first tissue. Then I applied the second one to her nose, and I said: "Now, let's give that nose a nice clean blow, shall we?" She did so, and then I used another tissue to wipe the few remaining traces from her face.

"Oh thank you so much," she murmured. "Thank you, thank you, thank you, thank you..."

Gradually, she stopped crying. And then, after a while, we started talking. I don't remember exactly how we got on to talking about her case, but it was only natural that we should discuss it. After all, it was the reason why she was in this bloody hospital to begin with, wasn't it?

When Dorothy had stood trial, the main stumbling block in her defence had been that she had killed her husband while he had been asleep, and therefore, he couldn't defend himself. She explained to me that this had been the only chance that she'd had to do it. If she had tried to do it while he had been awake, he would easily have defeated her, and then he would have undoubtedly battered her some more in retaliation. At any rate, if she hadn't killed him in some way, he would probably have killed her one day, considering the way he behaved towards her. Not that he'd ever given any indication of any such thing to the rest of the world, though.

"He was always perfectly charming when we were in public," she said. "He was always the perfect gentleman, no one else knew what a beast he could be in private. He never let on to anyone else. But I knew, of course. After all, it was me who he was being a beast to."

I asked her why she hadn't simply left him. She said that she hadn't anywhere else to go to. She had no living relatives, or close friends. And even if her home life had become hell for her, it was still her home, after all. She hadn't got any other home to go to. I could understand all that. There were probably many battered women who were in the same situation that she had been in.

I asked her why she hadn't told anyone else about all this; why she hadn't gone to the police. After all, it was their job to deal with crime, and surely wife battering is a crime, if anything is. But even before she answered my question, I thought that I could guess the answer for myself, and as it turned out, I was right. There can be some forms of victimisation which the victim can find almost, if not totally, impossible to talk about. Frequently because of feelings of shame, I suppose, even if those feelings are totally unjustified. Or simply because it's too painful to describe the suffering in words. Victims of rape, for example, can have those problems. Victims of school bullying can have those problems. And victims of domestic abuse, such as wife battering, or child battering, can have those problems.

But of course, the question why Dorothy had not done certain things in the past, was all rather academic now. It didn't really affect the question of what could be done now. It seemed to me that the only solution was to find someone who knew that her husband had been a batterer, and could thus support Dorothy's claims.

"Surely there must be <u>someone</u> who knows the sort of man your husband was, Dorothy," I said. "Someone from his past; someone for his background."

She shook her head.

"Oh no, I don't think so," she said. "I think all of his relatives are dead. I don't know for sure, because he originally came from Australia, but I don't <u>think</u> any of them are still alive, now. Oh, there's his first wife, of course – but I'm not even sure if <u>she's</u> still alive, now."

This brought me up sharp.

"Are you saying he was married before?" I said. "You mean, in Australia?"

"Yes."

"Well, what happened to his first wife, then?"

"Oh, they split up."

"Do you have any idea why?"

"Oh no, he never said. He didn't like talking about it, and I didn't like to press him. Why? Do you think it's important?"

"Well, of course it is!" I exclaimed. "Don't you see? Why did they split up? Maybe he left her, but on the other hand, maybe she left him. And maybe she left him because he battered her. That could help your claims that he battered you!"

Dorothy's jaw dropped.

"Now why on earth didn't I think of that?" she cried. "How could I have been so stupid not to think of it before?"

"Do you know her name?" I asked.

"Mary, I think it was. Yes, that's right, Mary." Her face clouded over. "But I don't know whether she's still calling herself Mary Little. She may have gone back to using her maiden name, and if she did, I'm afraid I just don't know what it is. For all I know, she may have married again, and if she did, I don't know what her new name is. And as I said, I don't know whether she's still alive, anyway."

"I don't suppose you ever met her did you?"

"Oh no, I've never seen her in my life. I've never been to Australia, and as far as I know, she's never been here. As far as I remember, I haven't even seen a photograph of her. I've no idea what she looks like at all. In fact, I wouldn't know her even if I passed her in the street." Suddenly, without warning, she started crying again. "Oh, I'd give anything to be able to walk down a street right now…"

I wiped away her tears with a clean tissue.

"Well, there must be some way of finding her, surely." I said. "What part of Australia did he come from?"

"Canberra. Well, I think it was Canberra. I'm sorry I can't give you an exact address. I'm not being very helpful, am I?"

"It doesn't matter, I'll find her for you!" I said. "I don't know how, but I'll track her down for you, somehow."

It was a rash promise, and I regretted saying it as soon as the words were out of my mouth. But I felt that I just had to say it. I had to say something to give Dorothy some hope. And it certainly have her some hope all right, Inspector. You should have seen the way her face lit up. It would have done your heart good.

"Then I'll be free!" she cried. "She can tell everyone how he used to batter her, and then they'll believe me!"

I felt that she was getting her hope too high. I had to bring her down to earth, somehow, in case things didn't turn out in the way that she wanted. That way, hopefully, the disappointment wouldn't be too great.

"Well, let's not get too excited, Dorothy," I said. "As you said, she may not still be alive. And even if she is still alive, she might not necessarily say what you want her to say. High might not have battered her, after all. Just because he did it to you, it doesn't necessarily mean that he must have done it to her as well."

A look of panic came into her eyes. There was no other way to describe it. I'd wanted to bring her down to earth. Well, I'd done that, all right. Only too well, I could have kicked myself.

"Oh, she must be alive, she simply must be!" she cried. "He must have battered her! She must back me up! I've got to get out of here. I've simply got to get out of here! You've seen that Senior Nurse. She's evil, that woman! She keeps on tormenting me. She says if I don't behave myself, and if I don't do exactly what she tells me, then I'll never be set free, and she'll have me sent to Broadmoor." She was beginning to get hysterical. "I can't go there. I've heard about the sorts of things that go on in places like that. I can't go there, I tell you. I'd sooner kill myself…"

"You mustn't do that!" I exclaimed, sharply. "Whatever happens, you mustn't do that! Do you understand me? Do you understand me?"

She nodded dumbly. My sudden change of mood had evidently startled her into silence.

Instantly, I felt ashamed of myself.

"Anyway," I went on, reverting to a gentler tone, "Rawsthorne's just trying to put the wind up you." (As soon as I said that, I realised what an unfortunate choice of phrase it was – considering exactly what it was that had originally led to Dorothy ending up in the seclusion room. However, she didn't seem to have noticed my gaffe). "*She* can't have you sent to Broadmoor. The doctor's the only one who's got the power to make a decision like that."

But inwardly, I had to admit that, for all practical purposes, Rawsthorne *could* do just exactly that. As I told you, Inspector, the doctor hardly ever visited the wards. As a result, most of the decisions, that he made about the patients, were based on what Rawsthorne told him about them.

I didn't tell Dorothy any of this, of course. I didn't want to make her feel worse that she already was. And I didn't tell her, either, that I didn't really have the foggiest notion how to go about finding her husband's first wife, assuming, of course, that she was still alive. The only people, that I thought would be able to do that, were the police. And I'm very sorry to disparage your profession, Inspector, but I didn't really think that the police would want to be bothered with any of all this. After all, the case was closed. Dorothy had been convicted. And the police wouldn't want to admit that they'd been wrong.

But now that I've come to see you, Inspector, can you find that woman? I know that it's only a slim chance. I know that the woman may not still be alive any longer. And even if she is, that man may not have actually have battered her, of course. But it's Dorothy's only chance. It's her only hope. Can you find that woman for her, Inspector? I'm not asking for me, I'm asking for Dorothy …

Chapter FOUR

Meanwhile, back at the hospital (as they might say, if all of this was only a story – I truly wish that it was, Inspector, but unfortunately, it isn't ...).

I decided that I simply wasn't going to stand for the way that Rawsthorne and her cronies had treated Dorothy; no, I was going to make a complaint about it. I decided to go and see the General Manager of the hospital and tell him about everything that had been happening. I knew that Rawsthorne and those other two nurses would deny everything that <u>had</u> been happening, both in the bathroom and at the seclusion room. But at least, in the case of the latter incident, there was a witness in the shape of Nurse Evans, She hadn't taken part in the victimisation of Dorothy. And I told you, Inspector, how disgusted she had looked. I felt sure that she would back me up.

With hindsight, I can see now that it would have been a lot better if I had spoken to Evans about all of this first, before going to talk to the General Manager. It could have saved me a lot of trouble. A <u>whole</u> lot of trouble...

****

It wasn't unit a few days later that I finally got the chance to speak to the General Manager, but I was eventually able to see him in his office.

"Yes, Brenda, what can I do for you?" he asked.

I started to tell him all about it. But gradually, I got the feeling that he didn't seem to be at all receptive to anything that I was saying. Quite the reverse, in fact.

I thought to myself: Oh, no! I don't think that he's annoyed at all about what's been happening to Dorothy. I think that he's only annoyed at me for telling him about it, because it gives him the responsibility of having to do something about it. Ideally, he'd just like to sweep all of it under the carpet, and forget about it.

But undaunted, I ploughed on. I stressed that Evans was a witness who could back me up about what had happened at the seclusion room. I finally came to a halt.

He said that he would look into it. I left his office.

Because of the way that he had reacted to my complaints, I wasn't really expecting to hear anything more from him, to be honest. But as it turned out, I was wrong about that.

In fact, it was the next day that he summoned me back to his office.

"Ah, Nurse Dalton," he said, as soon as I had come in.

Immediately, I thought to myself: Oh, no! it looks like I'm going to be in trouble, here. The last time that I was in here, he called me Brenda. But now, he's calling me Nurse Dalton. That sounds distinctly less friendly to my ears…

"I've been investigating both of these allegations which you made, when you came to see me yesterday. First of all, about the incident which you say took place in the bathroom. I've spoken to all of the nurses who were present on that occasion, and I have to tell you that all of them deny your accusations totally. It's true that Dorothy Little became violent, and that, unfortunately, she had to be restrained and secluded, (she was released from the seclusion room a few hours later, as I'm sure you'll be glad to hear), but they absolutely deny that they did anything at all to provoke her into being violent in the first place."

Oh well, I thought to myself, I had been expecting something like that. I hadn't seriously expected Rawsthorne and those others to admit that they had done anything wrong.

"Now, turning to your other allegation," he went on. "This business about what you say went on at the seclusion room. Well, once again, I've spoken to all of the nurse who you named, and once again, they all deny that any such incident took place at the seclusion room at all." He paused briefly and then he added his killer punch. "And that includes Nurse Evans. You said that she would back up your claim. Well, I have to tell you – she didn't."

Well naturally, as you can imagine, Inspector, I was totally taken aback by all of this.

"What?" I exclaimed. "But she was there. She saw it all happen. And she heard it all happen. She can't just turn round now, and deny all of it..."

With a suddenness that made me jump, he banged his fist on the table. Loudly.

"Now, look here," he exclaimed angrily, "I've got enough work to do in this hospital as it is, without having to be bothered by malicious troublemakers like you as well. If you seriously want to qualify as a Registered Mental Nurse, at the end of your course, then let me tell you that you'd better watch your step. Now get out of my office."

I started to leave, but just as I was doing so, a thought occurred to me.

"But what about Dorothy Little herself." I asked. "She could confirm everything I've been telling you. After all, it was her who all of these things were happening to."

"Now, her word wouldn't carry very much weight, would it?" he retorted. "after all, she's mentally ill. Otherwise, she wouldn't be in this hospital to begin with, would she? Now, stop arguing with me and get out!"

I left. I was feeling furious with him, and I was also feeling furious with Rawsthorne and her cronies. But most of all, I was feeling furious with Evans. I was determined to have it out with her, the first chance that I got.

As it turned out, that chance wasn't very long in coming. Luckily, that day, Evans and I both went off duty at the same time. So I was ready and waiting for her as soon as she had left the hospital grounds. She saw me standing there. Obviously guessing that I was to talk to her – and obviously guessing, also, what it was that I was to talk to her about – she tried to avoid me. But as you can guess, Inspector, I wasn't having any of that. I walked straight up to her.

"I want to talk to you, Evans" I said.

"Well, I'm very sorry, Dalton, but I haven't got the time, right now," she said, and tried to push past me as she spoke. "I've got to get home to my family."

"Well, I'm very sorry too, but you're going to make the time!" I exclaimed blocking her path as I spoke. "Why the hell didn't you back me up when the General Manager asked you if you could confirm what I said about Dorothy Little? You saw what happened at the seclusion room, just the same as I did. And you looked as disgusted as I felt. So why, why, why did you lie about it? Why did you say that nothing had happened at all? Well?"

She didn't answer, though I must say that she did at least have the grace to look a little bit sheepish.

"Come on, tell me, I want to know!" I persisted.

"All right," she said at last. "Let's go somewhere and talk."

"Thank you," I said. "There's a café down the road. Come on, I'll buy you a cup of coffee."

****

A little while later, we sat in the café, drinking our coffee.

"All right," I said "Now level with me, Evans. Why didn't you back me up about what happened to Dorothy Little?"

She paused for a moment, and then, quite out of the blue, she said: "Are you married, Dalton?"

As you can imagined, Inspector, this was absolutely the last thing I had been expecting her to say.

"Evans, just what the hell has that got to do with what we're talking about, here – or with anything else, if it comes to that?" I said, in surprise.

"<u>Are you married</u>?" she persisted.

"No."

"Are you living with anyone?"

"No."

"Do you have any children?"

"No. But what –"

"Do you have any dependants at all?"

"No. Both of my parents are dead, and I was an only child." (Just like Dorothy, I thought to myself).

"Well, me, I've got a husband and three kids," said Evans. "And my husband lost his job when he was made redundant last year. My job is the only thing they've got to depend on. I simply can't afford to do anything that could put it at risk. If I try to make any trouble for Rawsthorne and her pals, then you can take it from me that *she'll* make trouble for *me*. Either she'll find some excuse to get me the sack, or else she'll make so much trouble for me that I'll want to leave, anyway. There are other nurses who don't like the things Rawsthorne does, any more than I do, but *they've* also got families who are dependent on them, so *they* don't dare do anything about it, either. I'm sorry to disappoint you, but that's the way it is."

I opened my mouth to reply – and then I realised there really *wasn't* any reply that I could make to all of that.

It was probably the same in many other jobs, and not just nursing, I thought to myself. There were probably lots of people who knew of all sorts of malpractices and abusers going on, but they weren't able to say or do anything about them, much for the same reasons as those that had been mentioned by Evans…

"Does Rawsthorne go in for this sort of victimisation very often, Evans?" I asked.

She shrugged her shoulders.

"I suppose it really depends on the sort of opportunities she gets. Obviously, she couldn't do those sorts of things to the voluntary patients. They'd just leave, and make a complaint to someone. And she wouldn't do things like that to all of the committed patients, either. There wouldn't be any fun in doing those things to those committed old biddies on the psychiatric ward, for example. They're so far gone that they wouldn't really be capable of suffering, anyway. They wouldn't really be capable of knowing what it was that Rawsthorne was doing to them, and they're also so far gone that they're never going to leave the hospital, anyway. So Rawsthorne couldn't make them do what she wanted by threatening to lock them up forever, because they're already going to remain locked up forever, anyway."

Evans was just confirming all the things that I had already deduced for myself.

"But obviously, we do get other kinds of committed patients, sometimes" she went on "Ones who do know what's going on around them, who are capable of suffering, who do want to get out, and will do almost anything, or put up with almost anything, in order to be released one day. Of course, it wouldn't be a good idea for Rawsthorne to do any of those things to a committed patient who had a lot of visitors, because the patient might complain to them, and then they might complain to someone else in turn. But once in a while, you'll get a committed patient who doesn't get any visitors at all; someone all alone in the world; someone totally helpless, in effect…."

Once again, all of this was just a confirmation of all of the things that I had already managed to work out for myself.

"You mean, someone like Dorothy Little, in fact," I said.

"Yes, someone just like her. But, as I said, there have been others in the past. Others who have had to put up with all sorts of things, in order to get out of the place."

"But surely, some of them would complain to someone else about those things, once they had got out?" I asked.

Evans shook her head. "Oh no, they wouldn't."

"But why on earth not?" I said in surprise.

"Just thing about it for a minute, Dalton," said Evans, patiently. "If they complained, they could be diagnosed as suffering from paranoid delusions. They might get put back in the hospital again. They'd be only too glad to have got out of the place. And they wouldn't want to jeopardise that, in any way."

"Well," I said, "at any rate, all of them did eventually get out of that place, didn't they?"

"Oh yes," said Evans, "they all got out ... well, in one way or another."

"Just what do you mean by that, Evans?" I said sharply. "Why did you say it in that way?"

Evans paused for a moment before replying. "I'm afraid one of them only got out of the hospital in a wooden box," she said at last. "One of them killed herself. She slashed her wrists. And to this day, I still don't know how she managed to do it. After all, they're supposed to keep all sharp objects away from the committed patients, in order to stop them from hurting themselves, or hurting other people. But somehow, don't ask me how, she did it. It seems that Rawsthorne had pushed her just too far."

"Well, please tell me about it, Evans," I said. "I might as well know everything Rawsthorne is capable of."

“Well, I warn you it’s not a very pleasant story,” said Evans.

“Do you know, I don’t imagine it would be, somehow,” I responded, dryly.

Chapter FIVE

"Would you mind if I stopped for a few minutes, Inspector?" asked Brenda. "It's all of this talking. It's making my mouth rather dry."

"It sounds to me like you could do with another coffee," said the Inspector.

"Oh, thank you very much – that is, if you're sure it's not too much trouble…"

"Oh no, it's perfectly all right. Could you remind me how you take it, though – I'm afraid I've forgotten…"

"White, with two sugars, please."

After the coffee had arrived, and while Brenda was drinking it, the Inspector said: "You know, Ms. Dalton, everything you've been telling me so far is all very interesting – I would have to admit it's all very disturbing, as well. But I have to tell you that so far, I don't think any of it is really a matter for the police. It's really a matter for the health authorities, instead."

"Well, I haven't finished yet, Inspector," said Brenda. "There's still a lot more to come. And I think some of it really is a matter for the police. So if you could just bear with me…"

As soon as Brenda had finished her coffee, the Inspector said: "Are you ready to go on, now?"

"Yes, thanks. Well anyway, Inspector – to get back to what Evans was telling me, about this patient who killed herself…"

Chapter SIX

It was quite a tale that she had to tell to me, Inspector. And it is quite a tale for me to have to repeat to you now.

I don't know if, by any chance, you remember the Pattie Stephens case, do you? Well, it was some years ago now, but it was in all the local papers, at the time that it happened. Pattie Stephens was a schoolgirl who was committed to the hospital after she had made a knife attack on a fellow pupil. It happened during the school dinner time break, one day. As luck would have it, all the older girls including Pattie, were allowed to use real knives to eat with; while, be contrast, all the younger girls (it was an all girls' school, by the way) were only allowed to use plastic ones. If only Pattie had been a few years younger, at the time, then perhaps nothing would have happened that did happen, that day.

When it occurred, a lot of the witnesses (teachers, pupils and dinner ladies) would describe later on the enormous shock that they all got on that occasion, one moment, Pattie seemed to be sitting there quietly, eating her dinner just like everyone else. (Though some witnesses would later say that there seemed to be a peculiar expression on her face). Then suddenly, without any warning, she let out an ear-piercing scream, and she launched herself, dinner knife in hand, on another girl. She slashed at her face, again and again and again. And all the time that she was doing it, she continued to scream her loud, penetrating scream.

Now, everyone was so taken aback by this, that it was actually quite a while before anyone thought of reacting to it. Then finally, three teachers and a dinner lady ran forward in order to restrain Pattie. But the delay had given her enough time to cut the other girl's face pretty badly. And later, it was declared a miracle that the other girl's eyes had escaped without injury. However, some of the knife marks would remain on her face for the rest of her life, according to the doctors.

The four adults managed, gradually, to pull Pattie off of the other girl, and they also managed to wrest the knife from her hand. (Though in the process, one of the teachers unfortunately got a cup across her knuckles). Following this, they managed to grab an arm or leg apiece, and then between them, the four of them carried the kicking, struggling, screaming girl out of the dining hall. Her screams gradually faded away into the distance, although they still seemed to echo in many people's ears for a little while afterwards. And she had certainly left plenty of evidence of her outburst in her wake. Chairs had been overturned; dinner plates and their contents had been knocked to the floor; water jugs had been overturned and their contents had been split.

It was discovered, after Pattie's eventual death – when it was too late, of course, for the discovery to be of any good to her – that her outburst had in fact been the final result of the cumulative effect of prolonged bullying by other girls, including the one whom she attacked. It seemed that previously, Pattie had been too inhibited to retaliate in any way. She was one of those mousy little girls who would probably have found it too difficult, either physically or psychologically, to retaliate anyway. (The bullies had obviously taken advantage of this; but then, bullies are usually too cowardly to pick on someone their own size). But clearly, it ha all been building up inside her for quite some time; so that when she eventually snapped, it was like a dam which had suddenly burst, after the pile of water had finally made the pressure just too great to bear any longer.

She was committed to the hospital, where she was put in the locked ward. If only it had been another hospital, then maybe it could have come as a blessed relief to her, after everything that she ha had to put up with, at the school. But in order for that to happen, of course, the locked ward would have to be run by someone other than Senior Nurse Rawsthorne...

"Pattie Stephens was absolutely perfect for Rawsthorne's purposes," said Evans. "Pattie never had any visitors, you see."

"She never had any visitors?" I echoed, in surprise. "None at all? But what about her mum and dad? Surely <u>they</u> came to see her, didn't they?"

"Well, her father had died some years before. Her mother had married again, but Pattie's stepfather persuaded her mother that it would be better if they didn't go to visit Pattie. He was trying to get promotion at his job, you see. And he thought it would spoil his chances if he was associated with a committed mental patient, especially one whose case had been featured in all the local papers."

Just the same as Dorothy's so-called friends, I thought to myself.

"But surely her mother could have come to visit Pattie on her own!" I said. "Surely she didn't have any worries about being associated with Pattie, did she? It was her own daughter, after all!"

Evans shook her head. "From what I heard, Pattie's mother always did what the stepfather told her. It seems she was one of those women who could be easily dominated. I suppose that's where Pattie got her mousiness from. And I father that Pattie and her stepfather had never got on with each other. He'd never really liked her, so they say."

"Didn't Pattie have any brothers or sisters who could have gone to visit her?"

"No, she was an only child." (Again, just like Dorothy, I thought to myself).

"Well what about friends?" I asked. "Did Pattie have any school friends?"

"From what I recall, she only really had one friend at school," said Evans, after thinking for a moment. "I don't know her name. Apparently, it was another girl who was always being bullied. It brought them together; not surprising, really. But after Pattie was committed, it seems the other girl's parents wouldn't let her go to visit Pattie in hospital. I assume they thought it would be harmful to their daughter, in some way."

"That girl's parents sound to me to be just the same as Pattie's stepfather," I said. "Well, anyway, what did Rawsthorne do to Pattie, if I dare ask?"

"Well, you name it, she did it," said Evans. "As soon as Pattie was admitted, Rawsthorne said to her: 'Now, just you get one thing straight, right away, my girl. I'm the one who runs things around here, not the doctor. I'm the one who decides when you'll be released – or if you ever will be, at all. The doctor may be the one who officially makes the decisions – but he does so, on the basis of what I tell him about the patients here. So you'd better behave yourself and do exactly what I tell you, if you ever want to get out of here.'"

"What a bastard. What an evil, gloating bastard," I breathed.

"Oh, but that was just the beginning," Evans continued. "She made Pattie always address her as 'Ms. Rawsthorne', just like the way you heard her make Dorothy Little do it. Rawsthorne made Pattie do all sorts of menial chores, like scrubbing the floor. She sometimes made Pattie clean the bath with a toothbrush – Pattie's <u>own</u> toothbrush. Rawsthorne, and those other nurses in her clique, would make fun of Pattie at bath times, like you saw her do with Dorothy. Rawsthorne would provoke Pattie, make her lash out, and then use that as an excuse to put her in a straitjacket and lock her in the seclusion room."

"Again, just like she did with Dorothy," I interjected.

"Yes. But she capped it all by threatening to have Pattie sent to Broadmoor, or one of those other high security mental hospitals. She got her into a real panic about it. In the end, Pattie took another way out – the <u>only</u> other way, in fact."

Evans paused, while she took another sip of coffee.

"Actually," she continued, after a little while, "I was the one who found her body. She was in the seclusion room at the time, but she wasn't in a straitjacket. If only she <u>had</u> been, then she wouldn't have been able to do to herself what she did do. I've never forgotten it, and I don't think I ever will. She was huddled in a corner of the room. There was blood splashed all around her. And, to make matters worse, Pattie's mother died, shortly afterwards – apparently out of grief over Pattie."

For a while, I sat silently, while I slowly digested everything that Evans had just told to me.

Finally, I said angrily: "And you admit you knew about everything that Rawsthorne was doing to Pattie Stephens, and yet you did nothing at all about it? You just let it all happen? You did nothing at all to help Pattie? And after Pattie died, you didn't inform anyone in authority about what you knew?"

"Now look, Dalton, we've already been all over that, in regard to Dorothy Little," said Evans. "Please don't bring it all up again, I beg of you. And I think that it's only fair I should tell you, that if you repeat any of the things which I've been telling to you, then I'll deny I ever said them. It'd be your word against mine. You haven't got any witnesses. I'm sorry, but I just don't want to get involved in any of all this."

"Oh, all right," I said. "But what a rotten break for the poor girl. Or rather, what a series of rotten breaks. If only she hadn't been bullied at school; or if only someone had stopped it, before it got to he stage where she attacked that other girl; or if only she had had a hospital visitor who she could have complained to, about everything Rawsthorne was doing to her..."

We sat in silence for a few moments.

Finally, I said: “Just why the hell is Rawsthorne the way she is, Evans?”

The shocking impact of her reply was, if anything, made even more startling by the matter-of-fact way in which she said it.

“Why is Rawsthorne the way she is? Well, I suppose, it’s for the same reasons you can find bullies and sadists among nurses in mental hospitals all round the country – and probably all round the rest of the world,” she said.

Chapter SEVEN

"What?" I exclaimed. I was totally taken aback by all of this. "What? You can't really mean that, can you, Evans? Surely, Rawsthorne must be some horrible freak of nature! There can't possibly be monsters like her among the nurses in every mental hospital in this country, let alone the rest of the world!"

"Now hold on, I didn't say there was someone like her in every mental hospital," she said. "I'm not even saying she's necessarily typical, thank God. In fact, I'm quite sure she's not. I'm just saying you can find people like her in a lot of those places."

"But where did you get this idea?" I asked. "How on earth do you know all this?"

She paused for a moment, while she drank some more of her coffee. Then she said: "How do I know? Well, mostly because of a book I once read. It gave accounts of various scandals and abuses that had taken place in mental hospitals in Britain over the previous twenty years or so. Rawsthorne's probably a saint, in comparison to some of the bastards in the book."

I snorted in derision. "Oh, pull the other one, Evans!" I scoffed.

"Oh believe me, it's true," she insisted. "I've read about nurses assaulting patients so badly that they died, and the nurses ended up being convicted of manslaughter. I've read about patients being sexually assaulted. It seems there was even one patient, once, who was used in a blue movie that the nurses were making for their own entertainment. When it comes to committing abuses against patients, those nurses could probably teach Rawsthorne a thing or two."

As you can imagine, Inspector, I was absolutely dumbfounded by everything that I was hearing.

"But what on earth makes people like this?" I asked.

"Partly the stress of the job, probably."

"Well, that's no excuse," I said. "After all, no one forced them to take on the job in the first place, did they? It was their choice. Besides, you said 'partly'. Are you saying there's another reason in addition to that?"

Evans shrugged her shoulders. "Oh well, you know what they say, don't you? All power corrupts. And absolute power corrupts absolutely. Let's face it, Dalton, most people don't usually have any sort of power at all, most of the time. They just go through the whole of their insignificant little lives, being total nobodies, total nonentities, total non-achievers. No one knows about them. They've not become famous for anything. If you suddenly put power in the hands of people like <u>them</u>, then heaven knows what sort of abuses they might commit. That's obviously the way it is, with Rawsthorne."

"But the *extent* to which she does it," I said. "It's just sadism. That's all it is; sheer, calculated sadism."

"Oh well," said Evans, shrugging her shoulders again, (it seemed to be a habit of hers), "I suppose we've all got a dark side to our nature, haven't we? I have. You have. We all have. I think Jung referred to it as the Shadow."

"Look, never mind about Jung and this Shadow of his," I said, impatiently. "The point is, we've got to do something about Rawsthorne."

Evans looked at me sharply.

"Look, Dalton, I don't know what the hell you mean by saying *we've* got to do something about Rawsthorne," she said. "Haven't I already told you why I don't want to get involved with any of all this? I would have wanted *you* not to get involved, either, if only you'd had the sense to come and talk to me before you went to see the General Manager. Oh well" – she shrugged her shoulders, characteristically – "I'm afraid it's all too late now. Rawsthorne will get her revenge on you for reporting her. Just you wait and see."

"Go on, let her do her worst, then," I said, defiantly. "I don't care. I can handle it."

Evans smiled, grimly. "Oh, you'll care, all right. There was something else I read about in that book I was telling you about. It wasn't only about the abuse of mental patients, you know; it was also about all of the nasty things that were done to whistleblowers like you."

"Oh? What sort of things are you referring to?" I said, nervously.

"Oh never you mind, you'll be finding it out for yourself, in good time," said Evans. "And now, I really must be going. My husband and kids will be wondering what on earth has happened to me." So saying, she got to her feet, and added: "Thanks for the coffee."

"Oh, just before you go, Evans -" I began.

"What the hell is it now?" she said, wearily.

"I'd like you to tell me the title of that book you've been talking about. And also the name of the author. I'd like to get hold of it myself, if I can."

She supplied me with the information that I wanted, and then she left.

There was one thing that I disagreed with Evans about. I didn't think that Rawsthorne had been corrupted by the power of her job. I thought that she had taken on the job in order to satisfy a lust for power which she already had!

And it wouldn't be too long, Inspector, before I would find myself on the receiving end of that same lust for power, myself…

Chapter EIGHT

I had hoped, Inspector, that Evans would turn out to be wrong about what she had said, regarding Rawsthorne getting her revenge. I had hoped that Evans was simply being melodramatic, or that she had just been trying to put the wind up me. But she was right. Boy, was she right! In fact, Rawsthorne started to get her revenge on me the very next day. I had expected her to give me a right good tongue lashing. We in fact, she didn't actually say anything to me at all. But she did put me to work on the female psychogeriatric ward, where I had to spend a lot of time cleaning up all those incontinent, elderly women. Take my tip and don't ever take on my job, if you know what's good for you, Inspector. Believe me, when you've wiped one bottom, you've wiped them all.

And those cronies of Rawsthorne's took their revenge on me as well. I was sent to Coventry. I was totally ignored, except for the purposes of work, and even then, they only spoke to me as little as possible; as little as thy needed to. Their only other contact with me was a physical one. They would "accidentally" bump into me; they would "accidentally" trip me up. It was all rather childish, really. You would surely have thought that grown adults would have had more maturity than that. But evidently not, it seems…

Now, you might at least have thought that when I went off duty, and went home to my flat, everything would be all right there. But even then, there was still a problem. By the way, Inspector, I suppose that you may be wondering how a mere student like me could afford her own flat? Well, I mentioned, earlier on, that both of my parents were dead. My father was a very successful businessman (by the way, have you ever heard of Gerald Dalton? Oh, you haven't) and he made a lot of money. When he died, the money passed to my mother, and when she died, it passed in turn to me. I was very glad to have that flat, because it meant that I didn't have to live on the hospital grounds. It was bad enough having to work alongside Rawsthorne and her cronies, without having to live alongside them as well. I was also able to afford a small second-hand car. I'll have more to say about my car a little later on...

Well, as I was saying, I even had a problem at my flat. It came in the form of an anonymous letter. It contained, in block capitals, the single word: BITCH. Well of course, by the time I'd unfolded the letter, and read it, my fingerprints were all over the letter and envelope, obscuring any others that might have been there. (Though I strongly suspect that they would have been careful enough to wear gloves at all times, anyway. And of course, the postman's fingerprints, on the envelope, would complicate matters as well). However, for what it's worth, I've kept both the letter and the envelope. They're at the flat, right now. When I get the chance, I'll give them to you, Inspector. They're evidence, after all...

Of course, if wasn't only the letter itself that was so worrying, but also the fact that they evidently knew where I lived. It made me wonder what <u>other</u> trouble I might have at my flat, later on...

Meanwhile, back at the hospital (to use that phrase once again!) things were about to come to a head – and as you'll soon see, Inspector, I mean that literally, as well as metaphorically...

****

I was down on my hands and knees, washing the floor in the female psychogeriatric ward (it was another unenjoyable task which I had been given to do) when Rawsthorne came in. I decided that it would be best just to ignore her, and carry on with what I was doing.

It was a few moments later that I heard her say: "You're slipping up, Dalton. You forgot to empty this."

I looked up, to see her holding up a bedpan, which was brimful of urine.

She was quite right, of course. I <u>had</u> slipped up. Emptying the bedpans was one of the first things that should be done each day, so that they could be used again as soon as possible. As you would have expected, they were much in demand in the female psychogeriatric ward.

"Oh no, don't trouble yourself," she said, as I started to get to my feet. "I'll do it myself."

I carried on washing the floor. I took my eyes off her. It was very unwise of me.

She emptied the bedpan, all right.

In fact, she emptied it all over my head.

You won't be surprised to learn, Inspector, that the sheer unexpectedness of it was enough to make me cry out in shock.

Luckily, the bedpan only contained urine, and nothing worse, though that was bad enough in itself. I just remained where I was. I was absolutely paralysed with shock.

"There, Dalton," she said. "So just what are you going to do about that, then?"

I knew, and she knew, that there was really nothing that I could do about it. If I were to make a complaint, and she denied it, it would just be my word against hers. There were no reliable witnesses, as the patients were all so confused and elderly in that particular ward.

For a moment, I thought of going straight to the General Manager, there and then, in my wet state. I knew that it would attract the amused glances of all the other nurses. But at least that way, I thought to myself, I would be able to back up my claim. But even then, I thought, Rawsthorne would probably claim that I had tipped the bedpan over myself, just so that I could then blame it on her. And if previous experience was anything to go by, I had the feeling that the General Manager would probably believe her (I wondered whether, by any chance, the two of them had got any kind of relationship going with each other. It might explain his reluctance to believe anything bad of her).

Rawsthorne started to walk out of the ward.

And it was then that I made a really big mistake. If only I had just said nothing, then she might have let it go at that. She might have felt that she had finally put this troublesome student in her place, and she might have been content to leave it at that.

But instead, fool that I was, I called out: "Why don't you go all the way and just kill me?" and then, before I could stop myself, I added: "Like you did to Pattie Stephens…"

She suddenly stopped sharp, as if she had been stung. And then she turned round slowly and walked up to me. I quickly got to my feel, as I did not want to be at any kind of disadvantage to her. We stood there, facing each other.

"I can see that Welsh bitch has been talking to you," she said. She meant Evans, of course. I mentally noted that Rawsthorne had used the word "bitch", the same word that had been in the anonymous letter. Not that I really needed any confirmation, of course, that she had been the one who had sent it. Who else could it have been, after all?

"Pattie Stephens killed herself," she said. "I didn't kill her. So don't you ever go around making accusations like that, Dalton. You could land yourself in a great deal of trouble."

I thought, but I didn't say: oh yes you did kill her, Rawsthorne. You and those school bullies between you – you killed her, all right.

Rawsthorne left the ward.

I felt very afraid at the time.

But believe me, it was nothing whatever, compared to the sheer terror that I would feel, later on...

****

Oh by the way, Inspector, I didn't tell you that I managed to get hold of a copy, from a library, of the book that Evans had been telling me about. And very disturbing reading it was too, as regards both the abuses of patients, and the victimisation of nurses who blew the whistle on those abuses. Evans had been right in what she had been saying. More and more, I was coming to regret that I had spoken out in the way that I had.

Incidentally, I don't suppose that it was only in mental hospitals that these sorts of abuses were happening, but also in other kinds of closed societies – such as prisons, and children's homes, and old people's homes…

****

And now, Inspector, we come to the events of today. It has, without doubt, been the most terrifying day of my life. I hope that I never ever have another one like it. Either of the things that happened to me today would have been terrifying enough on their own. But both of them, one after the other… well, it's a wonder to me that I'm in a fit state to tell you about them at all.

I had finished washing my hands after using the lavatory. (I seemed to be using it a lot. But that wasn't very surprising, really, when you consider just how tense the place had been making me, lately). Suddenly, in walked Rawsthorne, accompanied by those two other nurses. There was a key in the lock on the inside of the door. Rawsthorne turned it.

There were just the four of us in the room. Rawsthorne, those other two nurses, and me.

At a sign from Rawsthorne, the other two nurses walked up to me. One of them, a big woman got behind me, where she proceeded to twist my arms behind my back.

"Hey, what the hell do you think you're all doing?" I cried, in shock and anger.

But that was just as far as I managed to get, before the second produced a handkerchief and rammed it into my mouth.

And then I stared, in sheer disbelief and horror, as Rawsthorne produced, from an inside pocket of her uniform, a piece of broken broomstick.

"Get on with it," she said.

At which point, the second nurse proceeded to pull down my skirt and knickers…

Chapter NINE

No, I thought to myself, this isn't real. This can't be happening. This is only some horrible nightmare that I'm having. At any moment now, I'm going to wake up in bed. This just simply can't be happening. Rawsthorne's so high and mighty, that she probably thinks that she can walk on water. But even she can't possibly think that she could get away with…

Rawsthorne slowly walked up to me, and held the piece of broken broomstick just a few inches from my face. Then she continually looked back and forth between the piece of wood, and my exposed lower half, making sure that I understood the implied connection between those two things. I understood it, all right. In fact, I was so terrified that I urinated all down my leg. Even though I'd relieved myself only a short while ago, I suddenly seemed to have found a reserve supply from somewhere. I was incapable of feeling embarrassed about it. The only emotion that I was capable of feeling, right at that moment, was sheer terror.

For a time – which seemed like an eternity to me – it was almost as if all of us were frozen in some kind of tableau. Then, at long last, Rawsthorne said: "All right, that's enough." My arms were released, and the handkerchief was removed from my mouth. I collapsed in a heap on the ground, sobbing.

"That was just a warning, Dalton," said Rawsthorne. "Just to let you know we can do anything to you that we choose, and at any time we choose."

I didn't make any answer. I wasn't capable of doing so.

"And I wouldn't try making a complaint about this to the General Manager," Rawsthorne went on. "You haven't got any witnesses. It would just be your word against all of ours. And you weren't believed, the last time you claimed to him, were you? Oh, and while we're about it, we wouldn't advise you to rake up this Pattie Stephens business. It's all dead and buried, now."

Yes, just like Pattie is, you bastard, I thought.

"Now, why don't you do all of us – and yourself – a favour and just resign?" Rawsthorne finished. They made for the door.

Now of course, all of this had been the result of my last verbal outburst. So you probably wouldn't have thought, Inspector, that I'd dream of making another one. You probably wouldn't have thought that I could have been so reckless. But I just couldn't help it. I opened my mouth and screamed: "SCREW YOU, RAWSTHORNE! SCREW ALL OF YOU!"

They all stopped, and turned round. For one horrible moment, I thought that recent history was going to repeat itself, only that this time, it would be carried further – carried to the conclusion that I had been afraid it would be carried to, the first time.

But instead, Rawsthorne merely said: "Just cool it, will you, Dalton? Or else" – she held up the piece of wood, and in an unambiguous gesture, she pushed it up and down, several times – "it'll be you who gets screwed."

They left.

And then, some recent history did repeat itself.

For the second time, since I had started working in this hideous hospital, I felt the bile rise in my throat. I lacked the strength to get to my feet. Instead, with my skirt and knickers still round my ankles, I crawled on my hands and knees to the nearest toilet bowl. Once again, I only just made it in time.

Although I wouldn't have thought that it could have been possible, I was even sicker than I had been, the last time.

****

Oh well, I thought to myself (when, at long last, I had sufficiently recovered to be capable of thinking of anything at all) that's it. That really is it. I can't possibly fight against that sort of thing. I can't possibly fight against Rawsthorne and her cronies if they're prepared to go to *that* sort of length. So I'll just do as she says. I'll resign. I won't say anything to anyone just now. I'll just try to get through the rest of the day as best as I possibly can. Then I'll go home and I'll have, what I'm sure will be, the deepest sleep of my life. I reckon I'll need it. And tomorrow, I'll phone up and announce my resignation. I'll post back all my books and uniforms. That way, I'll never have to come back here, ever again.

And if nothing else had happened, Inspector, then that would have been that. I would have resigned (well, I'm going to resign, anyway, as I told you) but that's *all* that I would have done. Well, no *quite* all. I would have still tried to track down the first wife of Dorothy's husband. I wouldn't have just quit my job, and left Dorothy to the tender mercies of Rawsthorne and those other nurses, without making *some* attempt to help her. But I wouldn't have come to see you. I would have been only too grateful to get the wretched hospital out of my life for good.

But then, something else *did* happen.

I don't know whether they had planned it all along, or whether it was only because I had shouted at them what I did. Maybe they thought that my latest outburst showed that I was *still* defiant. Maybe they thought that I needed yet one more lesson.

But I still can't quite believe that they actually intended to kill me. Especially as other people could have been killed as well. I can't believe that they could have been <u>that</u> ruthless. I think that they just wanted to scare me into being silent about everything that had happened.

But instead, it had exactly the opposite effect. Which is why I'm here, now…

You remember, Inspector, that I told you, a little while back, that I had bought a second-hand car? It was only a small one – I could only afford to buy a small one – but it was enough for my purposes. Where I lived, you see, it was easier to get to the hospital by road, then it was by rail.

Well anyway, I don't know how I managed to get through the rest of today, but somehow I did. I was wondering if I'd be in a fit state to drive home. But when the time came, it turned out to be easier than I had expected. When I got in my car ad drove off, I felt as if a great weight had been lifted off me. I thought to myself: Well, I'll never see <u>that</u> place again, thank Christ.

My route home took me along the motorway for a few miles. I took advantage of this by picking up speed. I just wanted to get away from the hospital as quickly as possible.

I was driving down the inside lane of the motorway. I slowly increased my speed to seventy miles an hour. For the first time today, I felt able to relax.

I shouldn't have relaxed. I was tempting providence.

Because just then, all of a sudden, one of the tyres exploded.

****

Later, at the garage, they told me exactly what had happened. It seemed that part of the type had been cut out. It hadn't come out accidentally in any way; it had been cut out deliberately.

Now, at the time, of course, I didn't know exactly what had happened, or how. But somehow, even then, I knew that it wasn't an accident; I knew that they were responsible for it; that she was responsible for it.

But just then, of course, there was no time to dwell on any of that. I had lost control of the car, and I needed to regain that control. And fast.

Somehow, I managed to do so, and then my immediate aim was to stop. Thank Christ that I was driving down the inside lane at the time. It meant that the hard shoulder, where I could stop, was right next to be. I shudder to think what might have happened if I had been on one of the other lanes. I might have been killed (not to mention other motorists as well). And if I was dead, who would there have been to help Dorothy?

Anyway, I got on to the hard shoulder, and then I slammed on the brakes. I stopped so suddenly, that I'm sure I would have gone right through the windscreen if I hadn't been wearing my safety belt.

And that's when the reaction hit me, and his me really hard. I had a hysterical fit. I was wailing and screaming. It had all been welling up inside me for some time now: Dorothy, Pattie Stephens, the revenge tactics of Rawsthorne and her cronies, and now, finally, the events of today. If anyone had seen me just then, I would probably have been taken back to the hospital, only as a patient this time. (Just think how Rawsthorne and those other nurses would have licked their lips at that prospect!)

Gradually my hysterics dissolved into tears. I don't know how long I just sat there, slumped and sobbing. I seemed to have lost all sense of time.

Later it seemed years later, I stopped crying. Very slowly and unsteadily, I got out of the car, and set off to find the nearest phone. Luckily, I didn't have to walk too far; otherwise, I'm sure my legs would have given way beneath me. I called a local garage I knew, and they sent out a tow truck. When we finally got to the garage, they examined the tyre, and told me what I've just told you, Inspector. I left the car at the garage, but asked them not to repair it. I knew you would want to examine it for evidence.

Then I phoned for a cab. When it arrived, I told the driver to bring me here.

****

I'm sorry again about what happened in your reception area, Inspector. But as I told you at the start – and as I've been explaining to you, since then – I've been under a lot of strain, recently.

Well, that's my story, Inspector. So what happens now?

Chapter TEN

The great length of Brenda's statement, meant that there was quite a delay while it was being typed out. When it had finally been completed, Brenda read it and signed it. Then, the Inspector said: "You know, it's amazing. I think the whole thing's just incredible – nurses behaving like that. I thought it was supposed to be a caring profession. After all, they do call you angels."

Brenda laughed mirthlessly.

"If you asked me, I think it's more a case of dark angels, where Rawsthorne and her cronies are concerned," she said. "I don't know where they trained, but I don't think it could have been at any hospital being run by Florence Nightingale. Well anyway, as I was saying, Inspector, what happens now?"

"Well," he replied, "perhaps we'd better start by talking about what can be done for you, Ms. Dalton."

"Me?" said Brenda, in surprise.

"Yes, I was thinking that maybe you'd like us to give you some police protection, bearing in mind everything that's been happening to you, recently."

Brenda thought about this for a moment.

"Well, thanks very much, but please don't trouble yourselves about that," she said at last. "as I told you, earlier, I don't think they were really trying to kill me, but only to scare me. And when I phone them tomorrow, and tell them I'm not going back there, they'll know they've got what they want, anyway. I won't tell them I've spoken to you."

"Are you sure you don't want any protection?" the Inspector persisted.

"Yes, quite sure, thank you."

"All right, if that's what you want. Now, to the matter in hand. I think all of these incidents, which you've described to me, can be divided into three categories. First, there are the ones which the police can legitimately investigate. I'm thinking of the tempering with your car, and the hate mail. Second, there are the ones which we could investigate, in theory, but might have difficulty proving anything. I'm thinking, for example, of the time when Rawsthorne and those others attacked you in the lavatory. As Rawsthorne told you at the time, there weren't any witnesses to that assault. You do see he problem, there, don't you?"

"Yes, I see what you mean," replied Brenda. "But you believe me, don't you, Inspector?"

"Oh yes, I believe you, all right. As I say, the problem would be trying to prove it. The same goes for the time when Rawsthorne poured that, er, stuff on your head." (In spite of everything

Brenda was amused to notice how embarrassed the Inspector was). "You said the only witnesses, to the incident, were those elderly patients. And judging from what you told me, I gather they wouldn't exactly be the most reliable witnesses in the world."

"Yes, that's true enough," said Brenda. "Unfortunately, they're all so far gone in their senility, that either they wouldn't have been aware of what was going on in the first place, or if they were, they'd probably have forgotten all about it ten seconds later. Either way, there wouldn't be any point in trying to get any of them into the witness box.

"Third, and finally," resumed the Inspector, "there are all those ways in which you say Rawsthorne victimised Dorothy Little and other patients, including Pattie Stephens. Well of course, I'm as appalled as you are, about all of that. But I don't really think it's a matter for the police, but for the health authorities. I can only suggest you get on to <u>them</u>."

"What about Dorothy?" asked Brenda. "She's the one who I'm really concerned about. Can you track down her husband's first wife?"

"Well, of course, we've got contacts with police forces all round the world," said the Inspector. "Including Canberra. I'll get on to them for you. It shouldn't really be too difficult finding her, assuming she's still alive. But, as you said to Ms.

Little, she may not be. And even if she is, she may turn out not to have been battered by her husband, after all. And even if she was, Ms. Little wouldn't be released just like that. Her case would have to go back to the Appeal Court, first. It would all time some time."

"Yes, I know it's all a long shot," said Brenda. "But as I told you, Inspector, it's Dorothy's only chance."

She yawned.

"Christ, I'm really tired," she said. "I'm absolutely exhausted. I feel as if I could sleep forever."

"I'll arrange to have your car brought round here tomorrow, so that we can examine it for evidence," said the Inspector. "In the meantime, we'd better see about getting you home, Ms. Dalton. I'll tell you what, I'm just about to go off duty, myself. I've got my car here. I could give you a lift home, if you like. And when we get there, I can hang on while you get me the hate mail you got. Then I can start my investigations first thing tomorrow morning."

"Well, thanks very much." said Brenda. "It's nice of you to go to all that trouble."

****

They finally reached the block of flats where Brenda lived.

“Well, I’ll just pop upstairs and get that letter for you,” said Brenda.

“I could come up with you, if you like,” offered the Inspector. “That way, it would save you the trouble of coming down again, and going up again.”

“Oh no, that’s all right, thanks. I don’t mind. Just so long as I get the wretched thing out of my flat, that’s the main thing.”

“I’ll see you in a few minutes, then. Oh, by the way, please remember to bring down the envelope, as well as the letter.”

Brenda started to open the door.

“Oh, Ms. Dalton…” began the Inspector.

“Yes? And by the way, please don’t keep calling me Ms. Dalton, all the time. Just call me Brenda. Friends are usually on first name terms. And right at this moment, I feel as if you’re the only friend who I’ve got.”

“Well, it’s nice of you to say so. Well, anyway, Brenda - ” he stopped, not seeming to know how to continue.

“What is it?”

"Oh, I know I'm not a great one at making speeches, but I just wanted to say that I think you're a very brave woman. And a very compassionate one, as well."

"Thanks. It's nice of <u>you</u> to say <u>that</u>." Suddenly, impulsively, she leaned forward and kissed him.

"Thanks," he said, taken aback. "Why did you do that?"

"Because of what you just said. And as I said, just now, I feel, right at this moment, that you're the only friend who I've got."

She kissed him again. This time, he responded. Their arms went round each other. Then he undid her blouse and slipped his hand inside. He felt her nipple harden. He felt himself hardening as well.

"You know, there's more room on the back seat," he said. "You don't have to go upstairs just yet, do you?"

****

Afterwards, Brenda said: "Well, I did tell you, didn't I, Inspector, that I'm strictly heterosexual. Oh, that reminds me – about Dorothy. You <u>are</u> going to help her, aren't you?"

"Well, I'll do my best, I promise you that."

"Thanks. Well, I'll go ad get that evidence for you."

"Are you sure you don't want me to come up with you?"

"Oh no, it's all right. I won't be very long."

****

Of course, Brenda thought to herself, as she walked up the several slights of stairs to her flat, (she lived on the top floor), there was on thing that she hadn't told the Inspector – or anyone else, for that matter ….

She hoped that the Inspector would be able to help Dorothy. It was the most important thing, right now. Indeed, it had become even more important than the thing which had impelled Brenda to take on the job at the hospital in the first place…

She finally reached the door of her flat. She was just about to open her bag and get her keys, when she saw that the door was already open. In fact, it had been forced open, by the method of breaking the lock. And the lights in the flat were on…

With a quickening of her heart, Brenda went in – and gasped.

The place had been almost totally wrecked.

And the wrecker was still there – and was in the process of adding the finishing touches...

Rawsthorne heard Brenda approaching. She looked round, glared in recognition, and went for Brenda.

The flat's main room, which was where the two of them were, had French type windows, which opened on to a little balcony. In the course of the ensuing struggle, Brenda and Rawsthorne ended up on the balcony. Rawsthorne had gained the advantage. She was pressing Brenda up against the railings, and was trying to push her over the balcony. Brenda was trying to resist, but Rawsthorne was the stronger woman of the two. Brenda knew that she had to think of something, and quickly, or else...

Unseen by Rawsthorne, Brenda managed, quietly and unobtrusively, to raise one of her feet. She then stamped it down, as hard as she could, on one of Rawsthorne's own feet. Rawsthorne howled in pain. She involuntarily loosened her grip on Brenda. It gave Brenda the chance that she needed. Instantly, she pushed Rawsthorne off of her, straightened up, and grabbed Rawsthorne, who was still writing in agony, and was thus unable to resist. Brenda whirled her round.

Their previous positions were now reversed. Brenda now had Rawsthorne backed up against the railings. In fact, Rawsthorne was hanging over the edge so far, that it was only Brenda's grip on her that was stopping her from falling to her death.

There was a look in Brenda's eyes which Rawsthorne found really frightening. It was the look of an avenging angel…

"I've got something to tell you, Rawsthorne." Said Brenda. "And you'd better listen very carefully, because it's the last thing you're ever going to hear. I already knew about Pattie Stephens, before Evans told me about her. Pattie was my friend. Do you remember – did you hear at the time – about Pattie's only school friend, another girl who was always being bullied, just like Pattie was?" Brenda saw the dawning look at realisation – and fear – on Rawsthorne's face. Brenda nodded her head, smiling. "Yes, that's right, Rawsthorne, that girl was me. That bullying drew Pattie and me to each other. We seemed to spend all of out time crying on each other's shoulders. I suppose I was lucky, really. I survived all that bullying. But Pattie didn't. You bastards killed her. Those bullies were the ones who started it, but you were the one who finished it. Maybe I could have helped her, but my mum and dad wouldn't let me go to visit her in that bloody place. You could have helped her – it was your job to, after all – but instead, you put her through hell. Those bullies had already put her through hell, and then you put her through more of it. Just like you've put Dorothy Little though hell, and other patients also. Well now, you're going to Hell, Rawsthorne." As Brenda spoke, she nodded he head at the ground below. "You're going all the way down to Hell..."

"No," Rawsthorne whimpered in terror. "Please..."

Brenda felt a savage joy, upon hearing Rawsthorne begging for mercy. It showed her up for the sort of coward that bullies like her were. Before Brenda's eyes, Rawsthorne's face seemed to dissolve and re-form into the faces of the bullies who had made life such hell for Pattie and Brenda at school...

"Yes, Rawsthorne," said Brenda, firmly.

She pushed Rawsthorne over the edge.

Rawsthorne screamed, and continued to scream, until she finally hit the ground.

****

Brenda heard footsteps come rushing up the stairs.

She couldn't and wouldn't say anything to anyone about Pattie, of course.

"My God," said the Inspector, as he rushed in. "What on earth happened here, then?"

"She tried to kill me," said Brenda. "She tried to push me over the balcony. But luckily, she lost her balance, and fell over, herself."

The Inspector peered over the balcony at Rawsthorne's body, as it lay on the ground far below.

"Oh well," Brenda went on "at any rate, it avoids the expense of a trial, doesn't it?"

"Are you all right, Brenda?"

"Oh yes. I'm all right – now."

"All the same, you know, you could have been killed," said the Inspector. "I should have come upstairs with you, like I offered to. I should have insisted on it."

"Oh, that's all right, Inspector," said Brenda. "That's perfectly all right."

And she meant it, too. If the Inspector had accompanies her upstairs he could indeed have protected her. But then, she wouldn't have had the chance to kill Rawsthorne...

****

Brenda sat in the bus, as it slowly journeyed up the hill, and reflected on everything that had happened.

When she had started work at the hospital, she hadn't really had any set course of action planned. She had wanted to see her friend's destroyer with her own eyes, but she hadn't been sure what would happen next. But she had been sure that something would happen. And it had. It certainly had...

She opened her bag, took out Dorothy's letter, and started to read it again.

Dearest Brenda,

I'm free! And it's all thanks to you. I can't possibly thank you enough. You were right! His first wife, bless her, was able to tell the Appeal Court all about how he continually beat her, until she couldn't stand it any more, and she let him. Thanks to her, and thanks to you, I'm out of that awful hospital for good.

From all that I've bee hearing, you've certainly changed a lot of things! As well as getting ride of that evil Rawsthorne woman for good (I wish that I'd been there to see her die) you got an enquiry made into all the goings on at the hospital. I heard that, as a result, those other nurses, in Rawsthorne's clique, have been sacked, an barred for life from ever working as nurses again. I also heard that the General Manager was forced to resign, for letting all those things go on under his nose. And finally, I heard that the hospital has been put under new management.

> But most of all, you set me free – you, and Inspector Donaldson. I can't imagine how I'll ever be able to repay you, Brenda, but if you think of anything, just let me know.
>
> All my love,
>
> Dorothy.

Everything had worked out just fine, Brenda thought to herself, as she put Dorothy's letter away again. Except for Pattie, of course. Brenda couldn't bring her back to life. She had managed to avenge her, but even the avenging was far from complete. It was true that Rawsthorne had got her comeuppance (or should that be a come<u>down</u>ance?) and it was also true that those other nurses had received a punishment of a sort. So had the General Manager. But those school bullies – the original culprits – had got off scot free. Brenda still felt guilty about not having been able to save Pattie. But at least she had been able to save Dorothy. It helped, in a little way, to ease her feelings of guilt about Pattie.

Indeed, it had stopped Brenda from suffering a double burden of guilt. When she had witnessed Rawsthorne victimising Dorothy, Brenda had had a mental picture of Rawsthorne doing the same sorts of things to Pattie. (It had really been for <u>that</u> reason – and not just the victimisation of Dorothy, cruel though it was – that Brenda had been physically sick, on that occasion). Having failed to rescues Pattie from Rawsthorne's clutches, Brenda knew that she simply had to rescue Dorothy. Otherwise, Brenda would have suffered an extra burden of guilt, which would have been just too much for her to bear. She had bee particularly worried when Dorothy had talked about killing herself. Brenda still felt a bit ashamed of herself for having responded to Dorothy so sharply, on that occasion. But if Dorothy had known, at the time, about Brenda and Pattie, then Brenda was sure that Dorothy would have understood the reason for Brenda's sharp response. After all, Brenda had taken on her job at the hospital, because of one suicide that had taken place. She hadn't wanted there to be another one as well...

****

Brenda got off the bus stop outside the cemetery.

She hadn't told anyone where she was going, of course. It was vital that no one should know about her connection with Pattie. It would have led to some very awkward questions...

She approached the grave. Under Pattie's name, birth date and death date, was the inscription: FINALLY AT PEACE.

Brenda knelt down and placed the wreath by the grave.

"Well, I killed Rawsthorne for you, Pattie," she said. "And one day, I'll track down and kill all those bullies from school as well. I'll start with the one you went for, in that dining hall..."

PART TWO

Chapter ELEVEN

Jane Browning restlessly tossed and turned in her sleep. She was having that same nightmare again. And it was a particularly horrific one, at that.

In it, she was back at her old school again; to be more precise, she was in the school dining hall. Pattie Stephens was attacking her with a knife, and while she was doing so, she was screaming at her. The knife was striking Jane's face, again and again and again.

It was a nightmare that she had been having quite of number of times lately…

It was just at that point that she finally woke up. After a little while, she managed to get her bearings, and then she thought to herself: Thank God that it was all just a bad dream. And thank God, too, that all of this Pattie Stephens business was all in the past, now. It was all behind her. It was all dead and buried – just like Pattie Stephens herself was, in fact…

And it was then, just at that moment, after she had finally been able to relax for the first time since she had woken up, that the door suddenly burst open, and the light was just as suddenly switched on.

The abrupt, unexpected brightness dazzled her. Involuntarily, she blinked her eyes in reaction to it.

When she could finally focus properly, she saw that there were two women standing over her bed.

She thought to herself that this must simply for a continuation of her nightmare, and that she only had to shut her eyes, and then to open them again, in order to make the women disappear. But after she had shut and re-opened her eyes, the women were still there. With a mounting sense of trepidation, she realised that this was no nightmare. No, this was for real…

"Who are you? How did you get in?" she cried. "What are you doing here? What do you want?"

"Come, come. Don't you know who I am, Browning?" said the shorter of the two women. "Just take closer look at me." As she spoke, she leant forward.

Browning took a closer look at her intruder – and gradually realised, with dawning horror, just who that intruder was. Her mouth gaped wide open.

"Dalton…" she breathed.

It seemed that all that Pattie Stephens business was not, after all, behind her; it was not all in the past; it was not dead and buried. Instead, it had all come back to haunt her.

She wondered whether those nightmares, that she had been having, had been an omen of things to come – and things that had finally arrived.

Brenda smiled.

"Long time no see, Browning. You remember me now, don't you? Though I don't think you know my friend, here. Well, I won't waste your time, or ours, by introducing you to her. After all, you won't be knowing her for very long.

"As I said just now, you remember me. Well, you ought to; after all, you made my life hell at school, often enough. And I'm sure you remember Pattie Stephens as well, don't you. You made <u>her</u> life hell at school, too; so much so, that she finally went over the edge, and attacked you in the dining hall. Of course, I was no longer at the school myself, by this time – things had got so bad for me – but I heard all about it. I can still see some of the marks, from Pattie's attack, on your face. Quite fitting, really, when you come to think of it. I feel they reflect your ugly personality."

Browning listened to all of this in stunned silence. She seemed to be incapable of saying anything.

"As you know," Brenda went on, "Pattie got out away in that mental hospital, off the motorway. But unfortunately, it didn't turn out to be any place of refuge for her. Quite the opposite, in fact. A nurse at the hospital bullied her to the point where she committed suicide. You know, now I come to think of it, you and that nurse would probably have got on together like a house on fire.

"Well, I dealt with that nurse… ah, I see from the look on your face, that you obviously remember reading about the hospital in the papers, when all the goings on there were exposed. As I say, I dealt with that nurse. And now, its your turn, Browning. You were always the worse of the lot at school. So I wanted to make sure you would be the first one I'd get my hands on. I've waited a very, very long time to do this. But it's been worth it.

"As I said, just now, you made Pattie's life hell at school. To take just one example out of many, do you remember the time when you put that plastic bag over her head? You almost suffocated her. She couldn't breathe. I suppose, when you come to think about it, that it's a bit like having a pillow pressed over your face…"

Realising the import of Brenda's words, and realising what was about to happen to her, Browning finally managed to regain her power of speech. She screamed: "No, Dalton! Please! I'm sorry…"

Unfortunately for her, it was actually the worst possible thing that she could have said, in those particular circumstances. At the sound of those last two words, a very nasty look formed on Breda's face. While the other woman grabbed Browning's arms, Brenda grabbed the pillow, and pressed it down on Browning's face. Browning struggled, but it was all to no avail. Her struggles gradually got feebler and feebler, and finally they ceased altogether.

Brenda continued to hold the pillow over Browning's face, until she was sure that Browning was dead.

Then, Brenda turned to the other woman, and said: "Do you know what, Dorothy? Right up to the last moment, I wasn't sure if I would be able to go through with it, when the time came. After all, killing isn't exactly the easiest thing in the world to do – even though I'd already killed Rawsthorne. But as it turned out, Browning made it a lot easier for me. The bitch signed her own death warrant – by saying she was sorry.

"Sorry! She wasn't the least bit sorry about what she'd done. If anything, she was only sorry about what was about to happen to her; she was only sorry for her wretched self."

"As I told her, I've waited a very long time for this particular day to come. But then, I didn't have anyone to help me kill her, until you came along, Dorothy. Still, they do say, don't they, that revenge is a dish best eaten cold. Come on, we'd better get out of here."

****

The police would not find any fingerprints; Brenda and Dorothy had been careful to wear gloves, at all times.

Chapter TWELVE

As soon as the two women were back at Brenda's flat, they broke open the champagne, they filled and clinked their glasses, and they drank.

"Well, we're definitely committed, now," said Brenda. Then, realising how the word "committed" could have unpleasant associations for Dorothy, Brenda blushed. "Oh, I'm sorry, Dorothy, I'll rephrase that and say we've done it now. Though I have to say I still feel guilty about dragging you into all of this."

"Now, look, Breda, you didn't drag me into anything I didn't want to be dragged into," Dorothy responded. "After all, I did say, in my letter to you, that if there was ever anything I could do for you, then I'd do it."

"But all of this is my quarrel, not yours…"

"I tell you, it's all right. I must say, it was lucky for both of us that Browning could afford to live in that big house, all by herself. We were able to force open that window at the back. If, say, she'd lived in a top floor flat, like I do – or like you do, here – it could have bee a lot more difficult for us to gain an entry, unobserved."

"Well, she came from a rich family," said Brenda. "All of us did, at our school. It was that kind of school. Here, let me give you some more champagne…"

****

A little while later, Brenda said: "Of course, you never knew Pattie, did you, Dorothy? I've got a photo of her. Would you like to take a look at it?"

"Yes, I'd love to."

Brenda rummaged in a drawer for a moment, and then she produced a battered old photograph, which she then handed to Dorothy. Dorothy took it and examined it. Pattie Stephens was a mousy looking girl with a pale expression of her face.

"You must have loved her very much to be doing all of this for her," Dorothy said, as she handed the photograph back to Brenda.

"We loved each other. Oh, it wasn't in any sexual way, you understand, just..."

"It's all right, I know what you mean."

"And in any case," Brenda went on, "I'm getting revenge for myself, as well as for Pattie. I was bullied too, don't forget. It finally got so bad that my mum and dad took me away from the school altogether. That was bad luck for Pattie, because it left her all on her own. We always used to go around together. That way, the bullies would sometimes – not always, but sometimes – leave us alone. But once I'd gone, of course, Pattie was all on her own – and accordingly, she was vulnerable to their attack."

"So you weren't actually at the school any longer when she attacked Browning in the dining hall?" said Dorothy. Then she clicked her fingers. "Oh yes, of course, I remember you said that to Browning."

"That's right. If only I <u>had</u> still been there, then maybe things wouldn't have got to the stage where Pattie lost control, and attacked Browning. And in that case, none of the rest of all this would have happened."

"But then, you wouldn't have gone to work in the hospital," said Dorothy. "In which case, you wouldn't have been able to help me. And that would have meant I wouldn't be a free person today. I know I'm just being selfish, but…"

"Oh, that's all right, don't mentioned it."

"No, I <u>want</u> to mention it. And besides, Brenda, it hasn't only been me who you've helped. As I said in my letter to you, the hospital has become a much more humane place now, thanks to you. None of the patients who are there, now or at any time in the future, should ever have to go through what I had to go through – or what Pattie had to go through…by the way, Brenda – have you decided who you want us to go after, next?"

Brenda smiled.

“Oh, I’ve been giving a good deal of thought to that question. Do you watch a lot of films, Dorothy? Well, have you ever noticed that the hero always kills the villains in ascending order of seniority? He always starts off with the underlings, and then he moves on to the second in command, and then, and only then, he kills the criminal mastermind himself – Mr. Big. I suppose it might make for a more exciting climax to the film, but I’ve always thought it’s being a bit silly, myself. After all, what if the hero got killed, or stopped in some other way, before he had finished what he set out to do? It would mean that the chief villain would get away with it, after all.”

“Well, I assure you that I’m not going to make that mistake. I’ve drawn up a list of all of those bullies. I’ve got all of their names, and I’ve found out all of their addresses. And I’ve listed them in what I consider to be descending order of evil. Not ascending, but descending. I started with Browning, because she was always the worst one of the lot. And besides, it was because of her pushing Pattie so far, that Pattie finally rounded on her, and then ended up in that bloody hospital. I’ve already decided which one it is I want to go after, next. Her name’s Pearson. Deborah Pearson. Apart from Browning, she was always the worst one of the lot. I’ve been doing some checking up on her, and on her habits. She lives on her own in a big house, too, just like Browning did. I know exactly the right time for us to break in. All of which makes her even <u>more</u> suitable to be the next one who we kill."

"But all of that's for another day. I don't want Pearson's death to come too soon after Browning's death, or else the police might spot the connection between them. So we'll leave it for a little while. For the time being, we'll give Pearson a stay of execution, so to speak. I'll give you a call, Dorothy, when I think the time is finally right for us to make our move."

"Anything you say, you're the boss," said Dorothy, she got to her feet. She yawned. "Well, it's getting very late, so I really think I'd better be getting off home, now. Thank you for a great evening, Brenda. I've really enjoyed it. Till the next time, then ...."

****

After Dorothy had left, Brenda contemplated Pattie's photograph for a little while.

Then she said: "First Rawsthorne, then Browning. I'm getting there, Pattie. Slowly, but surely, I am getting there."

She kissed the face on the photograph. Then she went to the drawer from where she had produced it, replaced it, and then she took out a sheet of paper.

It was a list of the names and the addresses, that she had mentioned to Dorothy, of all of the girls who had bullied Pattie and Brenda at school. At the top of the list was the name Jane Browning. Brenda crossed it off. She did so with relish. She then looked at the next name that was on the list: Deborah Pearson.

"Well, I don't know what it is you're doing right at this moment, Pearson, but whatever it is, you'd better make the most of it," said Brenda. "You've been living on borrowed time, all this while, ever since Pattie died. And now, your time is just about to run out..."

Chapter THIRTEEN

The phone rang. Dorothy picked up the receiver.

“Hello?” she said.

“Dorothy? It’s Brenda here.”

“Oh hello, Brenda, how are you?”

“I’m fine. How are you?”

“I’m fine too.”

“Look, I just rang to say that tonight’s the night – that is, if you still want to be part of all this.”

“Oh, I do. Besides, even if I do say so myself, Brenda, I really think you’re going to need my help. I don’t think you could do it all on your own.”

“The Pearson woman lives closer to me than she does to you, so I think we should start out from my place – and come back here afterwards. Can you be round here at ten o’clock tonight?”

“Sure.”

“I’ll see you at ten, then. Goodbye.”

“Goodbye, Brenda.”

****

Deborah Pearson was lying in her bath.

She always enjoyed having baths; she found them just as pleasurable as having sex. She felt the warm water washing round her clitoris. On a sudden impulse, she started to caress herself. She gradually reached climax, shuddering with pleasure as she did so. Then she lay back, and relaxed in the water.

And it was just at that moment, all of a sudden, that the door burst open. Brenda and Dorothy came in.

There really could not have been a greater contrast between the relaxed state that Pearson had previously been in, and the shock that she felt, as a result of the intrusion.

She screamed: "Who are you?"

"Tut tut. Don't <u>any</u> of you recognise me after all this time?" said Brenda. "I know it's been a long time, but all the same…". Just as she had done with Browning, Brenda leaned forward, so that Pearson could take a closer look at her.

"<u>Dalton</u>!"

"That's right. Turned up like a bad penny, haven't I? I won't waste any time reminding you what you did to me, Pearson; I'm here to talk about Pattie Stephens. You know all about how she died, don't you? Well, you're partly responsible for her death, because you were one of those who made her life such a misery at school. I'm going to make all of you pay for what you did to her. I started with Browning – ah, I can see you heard about her death as well. Yes, that was down to me. Well, now it's your turn.

"Just to take one example of all the things you did to Pattie: do you remember when you pushed her head down that toilet bowl, and then pulled the chain?" Brenda eyed the bath water in a meaningful way. "How would you like to have your head pushed into the water – only permanently this time?"

Realised what Brenda was getting at, Pearson screamed again. "No, please…."

Dorothy grabbed Pearson's arms, while Brenda pushed her head under. After a while, she brought Pearson to the surface, coughing and spluttering. She pushed Pearson's head under again, and then brought her to the surface again.

Brenda looked Pearson directly in the eye, with an expression that was totally without any trace of pity or mercy.

"Tell me, Pearson, do you know that old joke about putting your head in a buck of water three times, and taking it out twice?" she said. "Well, here's the punch line…"

She pushed Pearson's head under the water again. And this time, she kept it there.

Just as had been the case with Browning, Pearson's struggles gradually got feebler and feebler, and finally ceased altogether. But Brenda continued to keep the other woman's head under the water, until she was sure that Pearson was dead.

****

Once Brenda and Dorothy were back at Brenda's flat, they got out the champagne.

A little while later, Brenda said: "You know, Dorothy, there's a certain poetic justice about all of this I really like. Browning almost suffocated Pattie when she put that plastic bag over her head; well, we suffocated Browning in turn. Pearson pushed Pattie's head down that toilet bowl; well, in turn, we pushed Pearson's head into that bath water…oh, another thing, Dorothy, did you notice how both Browning and Pearson begged for mercy, or words to that effect? Rawsthorne was just the same on my balcony. Well, you know what they say, don't you: if you can't take it, you shouldn't dish it out. Well, these bastards sure know how to dish it out – but it seems they just haven't got the guts to take it…"

Chapter FOURTEEN

The team of police officers, who had been entrusted with investigating the murder of Deborah Pearson, were totally different from the team of police officer who had been put in charge of investigating the murder of Jane Browning.

Just as was the case with the Browning team, so, too, the Pearson team were not getting anywhere with their enquiries. They had not found any fingerprints at the scene of the crime; once again, Brenda and Dorothy had been very careful to wear gloves all of the time. The police could not discover any motive for the murder. And they could not find any witnesses who had seen anything. In short, they simply did not have any kind of lead at all.

And for a long time, no connections of any sort were made between the two cases. After all, on the face of it, there was no reason at all why any connection should be made between the two cases – especially when it was borne in mind that the methods of murder, that had been used, had been different in the two crimes.

And then, one day, just on a sudden impulse, and more out of desperation than for any other reason, Inspector Norman Jackson, the police officer who had been put in charge of the Pearson investigation, decided to feed all of the details of the case into the police computer that was known as the Home Office Large Majority Enquiry

System (referred to, for short, as the HOLMES computer).

Brenda had told Dorothy that she had wanted to leave a considerable gap in time between the murders of Browning and Pearson. This was in order to prevent the police from spotting any connection between the two crimes.

Or at any rate, Brenda had hoped that they would not spot any connection. But unfortunately for her, she had reckoned without the HOLMES computer (which was perhaps not very surprising really, considering that she was not aware that any such police computer even existed in the first place).

It was a computer that held within it the details of thousands of criminal cases, past and present. And it was possible to feed all of the details of a particular case into the computer, in order to see whether it had any features in common with any other case or cases. If it had, then it raised at least the possibility that the same criminals could be responsible for all of the crimes in questions. And in some way, that might just possibly help the police to catch them…

And now, Inspector Jackson, who was desperately trying to find any sort of lead at all in the case, was attempting to take advantage of the HOLMES computer himself. He was endeavouring to find out if, by any chance, it would yield up any connection of any sort, between the Pearson case, and any other case or cases, from the past or the present.

To be truthful, Inspector Jackson wasn't really feeling particularly hopeful. But then, when he read the printout from the computer, all of that suddenly changed. His face lit up.

"Bingo," he breathed, in triumph. "Jackpot!"

And with that, he hurriedly made his way to the office of his colleague, Inspector Desmond Greaves. He was the police officer who had been put in charge of the Browning case.

****

"Come in," said Greaves in answer to Jackson's knock. Jackson did so. "Oh hi, Norm. Take a seat". Jackson did so. "And how are you doing?"

"I'm fine. How about you, Desmond?"

"I'm fine, too. How's the Pearson case going?"

"Well, actually, that's why I'm here. How's the Browning case going?"

"Well, to be honest with you, it's not really going anywhere at the moment."

"Well, don't get too excited but I think I may just possibly have found a connection between our cases."

"Oh yes?" said Greaves, suddenly on the alert. "Come on, give!"

"Just on the off chance, I fed all of the details of the Pearson case into the HOLMES computer, to see if I could find a link with any other case. And it seems both Browning and Pearson went to the same school – that well-to-do girls' school, a few miles away."

"Hmm. Frankly, I don't think there's necessarily anything significant in that," said Greaves, dubiously. "Lots of women round this area went to that school, didn't they?"

"Ah, but there's more to it than that," persisted Jackson. "According to the computer, they were both in the same year – and in the same class as well."

Greaves whistled.

"Oh I see! So you think the killer may be someone who knew them at school? Someone who bore a grudge against them – and still bears a grudge now? Do you know, I think you could just possibly be on to something there, Norm."

"I'm going to go along and have a word with the headmistress at the school," said Jackson. "Do you want to come along?"

"Sure. It'll save you from having to tell me all about it afterwards."

"Of course, there may be absolutely nothing in it," said Jackson. "It could just all be a coincidence. We might be on a wild goose chase. But right now, it's the only damn lead we've got. Come on, let's get going..."

****

At one point, during the journey to the school, Greaves remarked: "You know, that was a bit of luck, that – I mean, the computer spotting that link between Browning and Pearson. I know it's a great computer, but I wouldn't have thought it would have spotted an obscure link like <u>that</u>."

"Well, the thing is," responded Jackson, "I couldn't find any motive for Pearson's murder. So I got my team to find out everything about her. And I mean <u>everything</u>. From the cradle to the grave. I ended up with a whole mountain of stuff. I knew ninety-nine per cent of it couldn't possibly be important. But then I decided to feed all of it into the computer, and hey presto. I remember it was Stanford who I asked to look into Pearson's school – and you know how pedantic <u>he</u> is about tiny details. I assume you did similar things, regarding Browning, and that's how the computer was able to come up with that link."

"Yeah," said Greaves. "I couldn't find any motive for her murder. So I – well, you can guess the rest…"

Chapter FIFTEEN

"Come in, gentlemen, please be seated. I'm Ms. Sanderson, the headmistress here. Would either of you care for a cup of tea?"

"Not for me, thanks," said Greaves.

"No thank you," said Jackson.

"Well, gentlemen, what exactly can I do for you?"

"We, that is, I, am investigating the murder of a woman named Deborah Pearson," said Jackson. "It happened a little while back now, but perhaps you may recall having read something about it in the local paper. I believe she used to be a pupil at this school."

"That is correct, Inspector. Do you believe it has something to do with what you're investigating?"

"Well, possibly/. My colleague here, Mr. Greaves, is investigating another murder – that of a local woman names Jane Browning. It was a few months before Ms. Pearson's murder, but you may perhaps recall hearing something about Ms. Browning's murder as well. We gather that <u>she</u> was also a pupil here. Not only that, but she was in the same year and the same class as Ms. Pearson."

"Yes, that is so."

"It's an interesting coincidence – that is, if it is a coincidence. But we have to consider the possibility that both murders could have been committed by the same person, and that the murderer is someone who knew both victims at this school – someone who bore a grudge against them. I know it's some time back now, but were you a teacher here, when those girls were pupils here? And if so, how well do you remember them?"

"Yes, gentlemen," Said Ms. Sanderson. "I was the headmistress here when Browning and Pearson were pupils here. And actually, I remember both of them very well indeed. Not to put too fine a point upon it, they were bullies."

Instantly, both men were on the alert. They exchanged glances.
"Oh really? You know, it could be a motive for the murders," said Jackson. "Would you happen to remember the name of any girl in particular who they bullied?"

"Well, the one who immediately springs to mind is Patricia Stephens."

"I seem to remember her name from somewhere," said Jackson, thoughtfully.

"You should do, Inspector. It was in the local paper at the time. Browning bullied her so much, that I the end, Patricia attacked her with a knife in the school dining hall. She, that is, Patricia, was put in hospital for it – that mental hospital, off the motorway."

"That reminds me that when I saw Browning's body, there were some scars on her face which were clearly old ones," said Greaves. "Do I take it they were caused by Patricia Stephens' attack?"

"Yes, that's right."

"I don't suppose, by any chance, you happen to know if Patricia is still in that hospital?" asked Greaves. "Or whether she was discharged at some stage?"
The headmistress shook her head.

"Whoever this killer is, who you're looking for, Inspector, I can tell you it's not Patricia Stephens."

"How can you be so sure?"

"Because she's dead."

"She's dead?" Greaves and Jackson echoed, simultaneously.

"Yes. She killed herself while she was in the hospital. She slashed her wrists."

"The killer could perhaps be someone who's trying to get revenge on Patricia's behalf," suggested Jackson. "Did she have many friends here at school?"

The headmistress shook her head again.

"As far as I recall, offhand, she didn't have any friends here," she said. "She was a shy, introverted girl – not the sort of girl who would make friends easily."

"But precisely the sort of girl who could be an easy target for any bullies?" suggested Greaves.

"Yes, I suppose so, now you come to mention it."

"What about her relatives?" asked Jackson. "Would you happen to know who her family consists of?"

"Well, she didn't have any brothers or sisters. And I know her mother's dead. She died, not long after Patricia did – as a result of grieving over Patricia. That only leaves Patricia's stepfather. And frankly, I wouldn't have thought he would have been all that bothered about Patricia's death, anyway."

"Oh? Why do you say so?"

"Well, it seems he and Patricia never got on very well with each other. He never visited her in hospital. He didn't want anyone to know he was connected in any way with a mental patient. Apparently, he was afraid it would affect his promotion prospects at work. And for the same reason, he wouldn't even permit Patricia's mother to go and see her, either."

"Well, he certainly sounds like a nice guy," said Greaves, sardonically. "Would you happen to have a record of his name and address, by any chance?"

"Yes. If you can wait for a few minutes, I'll ask the school secretary to get those details for you…."

****

As soon as the two men had received the information that they had asked for, they took their leave. As they did so, Jackson gave Ms. Sanderson the police station's phone number, and also his own extension number, so that she could call him f she happened to think of any more information which could be of use to them.

Chapter SIXTEEN

One their way back to the police station, Greaves said: “The hospital that Stephens girl was sent to – wasn’t there some scandal connected with the place? It was before I got transferred here, but I still heard about it, where I was. It was in all the papers, at the time.”

“Oh yes, there was a scandal there all right,” responded Jackson. “It seems the Senior Nurse there – Rawsthorne, her name was – was bullying some of the patients. None of the other nurses spoke out about it. Either they were too scared to, or else they were joining in with what Rawsthorne was doing, anyway. But eventually, a student nurse – I’ve forgotten her name, for the moment – did speak out, and as a result, got victimised for it by Rawsthorne and some of the other nurses. Then finally, she came to see us. She spoke to George Donaldson about it.”

“I remember it now, it’s all coming back to me,” said Greaves thoughtfully. “Didn’t it all end with the student having a confrontation in her flat with this Rawsthorne woman?”

“That’s right. After she’s spoken to George, he gave her a lift back home, so that she could give him some evidence she’d been keeping there. He waited in his car, while she went up to her flat. She found Rawsthorne up there, wrecking the place. Apparently, Rawsthorne tried to push her off the balcony, but Rawsthorne lost her balance and fell over herself, and was killed. The flat was on the top floor."

"You know, Norm, I wouldn't mind betting this Rawsthorne woman bullied the Stephens girl while she was a patient at the hospital, and that's why she killed herself," said Greaves. "She's already had to endure it at the school. It would be the final straw if Rawsthorne did it to her as well. Do you suppose it's got anything to do with what we're investigating?"

"Oh, I wouldn't have thought so," said Jackson. "As far as we know, Browning and Pearson were never at the hospital, either as nurses or as patients. No, it's the school we've got to focus on, not the hospital."

"Do you think this stepfather is the person who we're looking for?" asked Greaves. "Possibly not, if what that headmistress said about him is anything to go by."

"Well, we'll have a better idea about that after we've had a word with him," said Jackson. "But it's getting late, Desmond. Let's talk to him tomorrow."

"That's okay with me." Said Greaves.

But as it turned out, they never did get the chance to speak to him.

****

"Dorothy, I've decided who we're going to kill next," said Brenda.

"Who's it going to be this time, then?"

"Pattie's stepfather. He's as much to blame for her death as anyone is. He didn't go and see her in hospital, and he wouldn't let her mum go and see her, either. If they had gone, she could have told them what Rawsthorne was doing to her, and then they could have put a stop to it, somehow. And in effect, he's responsible for the death of Pattie's mum as well. She died, soon after Pattie did. It was all the grieving that did it."

"Where does he live?" asked Dorothy.

Brenda gave her the address,

"That's a lot closer to where I live than to where you do, Brenda," said Dorothy. "After it's all over, let's go back to my place. You can spend the night there, if you like. Oh by the way, exactly how are we going to kill him?"

"We're going to burn his house down. I've managed to get hold of a can of petrol."

"But Brenda, we can't walk thought the streets carrying a can of petrol. It would be rather conspicuous, to say the least. And everyone who saw us would remember us, after the fire had taken place."

"I wasn't suggested we walk there. You've got a car. Can you pick me up from my place and then drive us there?"
"Sure. You don't drive any more, then?"

No, I haven't felt able to, not since Rawsthorne sabotaged my car. You remember all of that, don't you? Even when the car had been repaired, I just didn't feel capable of getting behind the wheel. I ended up selling it..."

****

Gradually, the sound of crackling penetrated the man's consciousness as he lay asleep. He woke up – to be greeted by the sight of flames shooting up, just outside his bedroom window.

He leapt out of bed. Without stopping to put on any clothes in addition to the pyjamas that he was wearing, he rushed down the stairs, towards the front door. He opened it – only to be confronted by an impassable wall of fire, which forced him back inside. Without stopping to shut the door again, he rushed into the kitchen, where the back door was. He unbolted and opened it – only to discover yet more flames which allowed for no exit.

In a panic now, and again without stopping to shut the door, he made a frenzied examination of all the windows in the house, upstairs and downstairs. It was just the same with all of them, too. Each of them were totally surrounded by fire. Any attempt, to escape through them, would be impossible (and the upstairs windows were too high to jump from, anyway).

Help. He had to get help. Rushing into the hall, he snatched up the phone. But just as he reached it, it started to ring. He snatched up the receiver.

"This is for not helping Pattie when she needed you, you bastard," said a vaguely familiar female voice.

He banged the receiver down on the hook, and snatched it up again. But the voice was still there.

"I'm calling from a public phone box," said Brenda. "And I'm not hanging up. I'm leaving the phone off the hook. That way, you won't be able to phone out. You won't be able to dial 999. Burn, you bastard. You'll soon be burning in Hell."

He had made a fatal mistake in leaving the front and back doors open. The fire had gained entrance to the house, now. And it was spreading – it was coming towards him…

He had to get out, somehow. He rushed towards the front door again – and was engulfed by the flames.

Just before he died, he realised who his called had been – and he also realised the reason for him imminent death…

****

Jackson was awoken by the sound of the phone ringing. Sleepily, he reached out a hand for the receiver.

"Hello?"

"Norm? It's Desmond. It's about Patricia Stephens' stepfather."

Suddenly, Jackson was wide awake.

"What about him?"

"We won't be able to have a talk with him, now. He's dead. His house was burnt down tonight."

"Desmond, I notice you didn't say that his house burn down; you said that it <u>was</u> burnt down," said Jackson. "Are you telling me it was arson, then?"

"Oh, there' no doubt about it. Petrol was splashed all the way round the house, and was then set alight. They found the petrol can in the garden.

"I don't suppose that there were any fingerprints on it?"

"No. Whoever did it must have been wearing gloves..."

****

Back at Dorothy's flat, the two women heard an item on the local radio station's new programme, about the death of Pattie's stepfather. They hugged each other.

"We've done it" We've killed him!" cried Brenda. "This calls for some champagne…"

A little while later, Brenda said: "You know, Dorothy, there are some others who I'd like to kill, as well as the rest of those bullies. I'd like to kill those other nurses; the ones who were Rawsthorne's cronies. You know the ones who I mean. And I'd also like to kill the headmistress of my school. She knew all that bullying was going on, but she never did anything to stop it. But all that's for the future. Let's have some more champagne…"

"Brenda," said Dorothy, a little while later, "I've been meaning to ask you – how did you find out what Rawsthorne was doing to Pattie in the first place?"

"Well, I didn't know at first. But when Pattie died – I must have cried for about a week at that time – I thought it was odd. I'd thought that after everything that had happened to her at school, the hospital could have been a place of refuge for her – an asylum, in the proper sense of the word. But one day, I found out the truth, by pure chance. It was a few years later. I was sitting in the pub, and I overheard two women talking at the next table. One of them mentioned the hospital. I listened very carefully, without letting them know that I was doing so, of course. It seems one of the women had been a patient at the hospital, and Rawsthorne had given her a hard time. The other woman asked her why she didn't complain after she was released, and the first woman said she was afraid of getting put back inside again. (I remember Evans made the same point to me when we had that talk in the café, but that's by the way). Anyway., this woman went on to mention other patients who had been give a hard time by Rawsthorne. According to this woman, one of those patients was a schoolgirl. I just <u>knew</u> it had to be Pattie."

"Had you already decided to kill Rawsthorne, then, before you started working at the hospital"

"Well, I certainly did, after hearing everything that Evans told me."

"You're really serious about all this, aren't you Brenda? You really want to kill everyone who had any part in brining about Pattie's death."

"Yes, Dorothy, but there's no reason why you should get involved in this, any more than you already have. The longer we go on, the more risk there is of us getting caught. There's no reason why that should happen to you, as well as me."

"Oh no, that's all right, Brenda. I'll see this through with you to the end. If all those bullies were only half as bad as Rawsthorne was, I'll help you kill them with pleasure." Dorothy glanced at her watch. "Well, it's getting very late. I said you could spend the night here. The offer still holds..."

****

After he had concluded his phone conversation with Greaves, Jackson had tried to get back to sleep, but found he was unable to do so. He had the nagging feeling, at the back of his mind, that there was something they had overlooked. Something which could solve the whole case. Something which was right in front of their noses. But – just like the purloined letter in Edgar Allan Poe's famous story – it was precisely <u>because</u> it was in front of their noses, that he couldn't see it. Oh well, maybe it would come to him if he slept on it – providing he <u>could</u> get back to sleep...

Chapter SEVENTEEN

It was the following morning – the morning after the night before, so to speak. Greaves and Jackson were sitting in the latter's office.

Their mood could not exactly be described as a contended one – quite the opposite.

"First Jane Browning, then Deborah Pearson, and now the Stephens girl's stepfather," said Greaves. "Well, that settles it. Patricia Stephens is the motive, there's no doubt about it. Someone's out to get revenge for her death."

"But who?" said Jackson. "All her relatives are dead, now her stepfather's been murdered. And that headmistress said she hadn't had any friends at school. So who the hell is it?"

And it was just then, at that very moment, as if in answer to his question, that the phone started to ring.

Now, Inspector Jackson was not in any way a believer in telepathy or omens, or anything else for a supernatural or paranormal nature. He would have scoffed at the idea of any such things as those. But the phone ringing, just at that moment of all moments, gave him the eerie feeling, as he picked up the receiver, that this was going to be the breakthrough in the case that he had been looking for – a feeling that was intensified when he found out exactly who his caller was.

"Hello?...Yes, speaking..." he turned to Greaves, and mouthed silently: "It's that headmistress."

Greaves, too was suddenly on the alert.

"You have me your number, Inspector, so that I could call you if I thought of anything else that could be of any help to you. Well, I thought I'd better give you a ring, because I've just remembered something. I told you that Patricia Stephens hadn't had any friends at our school. But now I come to think of it, I remember there <u>was</u> one girl who she was friendly with. It was another girl who was often being bullied. I think the reason why I had previously forgotten about her, was because she was no longer at our school when Patricia attacked Jane Browning in the dining hall. The other girl's parents had previously withdrawn her from our school, when the bullying had got particularly bad."

"Can you tell me the name of this other girl, Ms. Sanderson?" asked Jackson. He managed to keep, out of his voice, his impatience over her long preamble.

"Yes, it's Dalton. Brenda Dalton."

"Would you happen to know what her current address is, by any chance?"

"No, I'm afraid not. I did ask out school secretary to check about that, because I thought you would want to know it. But it seems we haven't got a record of it. I'm sorry."

"Oh never mind, that's all right, we'll find Ms. Dalton, wherever she is," said Jackson. "Thank you very much, Ms. Sanderson, you've been very helpful. Goodbye."

He hung up the receiver, and then he related, to Greaves, the details of the conversation that h had just been having. Then he added, thoughtfully; "Brenda Dalton. Do you know, Desmond, I think her name rings a bell, somehow. Now, where have I heard it before?,,," suddenly, he stopped. His jaw dropped.

"What is it, Norm?" asked Greaves

"Oh…my…God…" Jackson said, slowly. He clicked his fingers.

"Brenda Dalton! That was the name of the student nurse who I was telling you about! The one who blew the whistle on Rawsthorne and those other nurses at the hospital! The one whose flat Rawsthorne broke into!" He got to his feet. "Come on, Desmond, let's go and see George Donaldson. He was the one who Dalton spoke to, when she came to see us."

"You know, Norm, it's a pity the Sanderson woman didn't think of Dalton when we spoke to her yesterday." Said Greaves, as he, too, rose to his feet. "If she had, then the Stephens girl's stepfather might still be alive, now."

"Well, if it comes to that, he might still be alive now, if we'd spoken to him yesterday," said Jackson. "If he knew about Dalton's friendship with his stepdaughter, he could have put us on to her. It was my fault we didn't speak to him. I said we should leave it until today, because it was getting late..."

****

A little while later, Greaves and Jackson were sitting in Inspector Donaldson's office. Donaldson looked on, while Greaves and Jackson read copies of the statement that Brenda had made to Donaldson on that fateful evening.

When both of them had finished, Greaves said: "Oh well, that settles it. Dalton is the one who we're after, there's no doubt about it. You notice she mentioned Stephens in her statement, but she doesn't say anything about having known her previously. She even quotes this nurse Evans as saying that Stephens had a friend at school, but Dalton doest say that she was her friend. The way she tells it, you would think the first time she had ever heard of Stephens was when Evans told her about her. Now, why should she keep quiet about knowing her, unless..."

He didn't feel that it was necessary to finish his question.

"All right, now, let's sum up what we've got here," said Jackson. "Stephens and Dalton are bullied at school by Browning and Pearson – and possibly by some of the other girls as well. Stephens finally goes over the edge, attacks Browning and then gets sent to the hospital. Rawsthorne then bullies her in turn; to the point, in fact, where Stephens kills herself. Dalton vows to get revenge. She gets a job at the hospital. We don't know, of course, exactly what plan of revenge it was that she may originally have had in mind. But as things turn out, she eventually gets the chance to kill Rawsthorne when the two of them have that fight in Dalton's flat. I think we can take it that Rawsthorne didn't lose her balance and fall over the balcony, as Dalton claims; Dalton pushed her over. Dalton then turns her attention to the bullies who started all of this off in the first place. She kills Browning and Pearson. Then she kills Stephens' stepfathers, who she probably considers to be partly responsible for Stephens' death. He never went to see her in hospital, remember. If he had, he could have stopped what Rawsthorne was doing to his stepdaughter. We'd better find out where Dalton lives, and round her up quick, before she goes after any of those other former schoolgirls... hey, hang on a minute, what am I talking about? You already know where she lives, don't you, George? You gave her a lift back home, that night. Give us the address, and we'll get round there sharpish."

“Would you mind if I came with you?” said Donaldson. “She knows me. That might make things a bit easier for her.”

“You mean, it might soften the blow a bit when we arrest her? Sure, you can come with us.”

****

At one point, during the car journey to Brenda’s flat, Greaves said: “Of course, it may be a bit difficult to prove Dalton murdered Rawsthorne. There shouldn’t be any difficulty with the other murders, but Rawsthorne’s a different matter. In theory, she could have died in the way Dalton says she did. You were there at the time, George; have you got any thought on the matter?”

“Well, I was sitting in my car with my widows closed,” said Donaldson. “So I didn’t see or hear what was happening on that balcony. I only heard Rawsthorne scream, and I saw her hit the ground. But to be honest with you, there was one thing that did puzzle me a bit at the time. Dalton said that Rawsthorne lost her balance, and fell over the balcony. In that case, she should surely have landed on her front. But instead, she landed on her back.”

“Oh well, that settles it, then” said Jackson. “Rawsthorne didn’t fall over the balcony. Dalton pushed her over.”

“Even if she did, I wouldn’t really blame her, you know,” said Donaldson. “It was probably self defence. Rawsthorne was probably trying to kill her."

"Maybe so," said Greaves. "But in all probability, Dalton would eventually have got round to killing Rawsthorne in any case. That must have been the reason why she took on the job at the hospital, to begin with. And besides, all those other deaths are definitely murders. There's no getting away from that."

"You know, Desmond, we really should have got on to Dalton before now," said Jackson. "I was mulling over the case last night. I had the feeling we'd overlooked something. Now I know what it was. We'd decided, hadn't we, that the killer was going after everyone who'd been responsible in any way for the Stephens girl's death. And although we hadn't read Dalton's statement at that stage, we'd heard enough, about all the goings on at the hospital, to assume that Rawsthorne had bullied Stephens there. That would have been enough to make the killer include Rawsthorne among his – or her – targets. Well then, we should have taken a closer look at Rawsthorne's death. That could have made us take a closer look, in turn, at Dalton. I remember, Desmond, you actually asked me if I though all that Rawsthorne business had anything to do with what we were investigating. And stupidly, I said no."

"Oh come on, Norm, don't knock yourself, don't put yourself down," Greaves protested. "Don't forget, the first we knew, about the connection between Browning and Pearson, was only yesterday. And we wouldn't have known about that, if you hadn't thought of using the HOLMES computer. I think we've made very good progress really, in the circumstances."

No more was said during the rest of the journey. Donaldson was rather glad about that, because he was not really in the mood for talking. He was, after all, on his way to arrest a woman with whom he had had a tender encounter in the back of his car. He would do his duty, of course, when the time came to apprehend her. But he was not looking forward to it. No, he was not looking forward to it at all...

Chapter EIGHTEEN

Donaldson, Greaves and Jackson had not received any response when they had knocked on Brenda's door. Now, they were all seated in the police car, outside the entrance of Brenda's flat block, while they planned their next move.

****

Having spend the night at Dorothy's flat, Brenda was returning home. She started to turn the corner into the road where her flat block was situated – and she saw the police car. Hastily, she turned round, ad started to go back the way whence she had come. And she did all of it so quickly, that one of the men, who were seated in the car, had been able to spot her.

****

"Well, she's not at home," said Greaves. "But she's bound to turn up at some time. Unless, of course, she knows we're on to her, and she's done a runner."

"I don't think she knows about us," said Jackson. "I don't see how she <u>could</u> know. As you say, Desmond, she'll turn up. We'd better get on to the station and get a patrol car round here to keep watch. That way, they can nab her when she finally <u>does</u> turn up."

Donaldson, who was sitting in the front passenger seat, relayed the request over the radio.

"I think we'd better hang on here, until the other car gets here," said Jackson. "Just in case she gets here before they do. And just on the off chance she <u>has</u> done a runner, as you suggested, Desmond, we'd better put out an alert for her. George, you've met her. You'd better get on to the station, and give them her description."

Again, Donaldson relayed the relevant message over the radio.

"You know, guys, I've been thinking," said Greaves. "I only saw the Browning woman when she was dead, but she looked a bit on the hefty side. It couldn't have been a very easy job for Dalton to kill her: especially not by putting a pillow over her face. Browning would surely have been bound to have put up a struggle."

"That's just what I was thinking about the Pearson woman, when I saw <u>her</u> body," said Jackson. "<u>She</u> was a bit on the heft side, too. Do you think Dalton had an accomplice, then/"

"Well, it certainly looks like it, doesn't it? But who could it be? I remember Dalton said I her statement that she didn't have any relatives. And we don't know who her friends are."

"Hey, wait a minute," said Donaldson. "What about Dorothy Little?"

"Who?" said Greaves, blankly. He had forgotten her name for the moment.

"You know," said Donaldson, "the patient who Dalton managed to get released form the hospital. The one who she spoke to me about. Little's probably feeling so grateful to Dalton, that she'd do almost anything for her. I'll get on to the station and ask them to find out what Little's current address is."

He proceeded to do so.

****

Dorothy opened the door in answer to Brenda's knock. She could tell at once, from the expression on Brenda's face, that something was wrong; that something was very, very wrong indeed.

"Brenda? I can see something's the matter; what is it? Why have you come back here?"

"Let me in, Dorothy, and I'll tell you."

****

"Guvner?" said the voice over the radio. "It's about he Dalton woman. A woman, answering her description, was seen entering the flat block in Depping Road. Over."

"Are they absolutely certain it's her?" asked Donaldson. "Over."

"Well, you know you wanted Dorothy Little's address? Well, that's where she lives. She's got a flat on the top floor." The radio voice went on to give them the number of the flat.

"Thanks a lot," said Donaldson. "Over and out."

Jackson tapped the police driver on the should. "You've got the address, son. Let's go. And sound your siren. We don't want any traffic to delay us. We've got to get round there <u>fast</u>, before Dalton and Little go off and kill someone else."

As they sped off on their way, Donaldson said: "You know guys, I really cant help feeling sorry for Dalton – I mean, when you consider why she's doing it."

"Well, maybe I feel a bit sorry for her, too," responded Jackson. "But she's still got to be stopped, hasn't she? We cant have her going around, killing people."

"Oh, I know," said Donaldson. "But when we arrest her – I know its not really my case, strictly speaking – but I'd rather you let <u>me</u> handle it, if you don't mind."

"No, that's all right with me," said Jackson.

"Me, too," added Greaves.

"And," Donaldson went on, "let's not forget how she managed to reform that hospital. The woman's become a local heroine..."

Chapter NINETEEN

"You can't just run away, Brenda," said Dorothy. "You've got to go back and face those policemen. You've just got to bluff it out. They might suspect it's you, but they don't know it's you. But they will do, if you run away."

"Yes, of course, you're right, Dorothy," said Brenda. "Though this means, unfortunately, that we won't be able, now, to kill any of those other bastards." She smiled ruefully. "It's a pity, that. It's just as well I thought of starting with the worst ones, and working my way down from there. I would really have hated it if Browning and Pearson had got away with it. And I'm glad we got that bloody stepfather of Pattie's. Oh well, suppose I'd better be getting back home…"

It was just at that moment, that they heard the sound of the approaching siren. Both of them rushed to the window and stared out. They saw the police car as it pulled up outside the block of flats.

"It looks like you were right, Brenda," said Dorothy, heavily, as the two of them turned away from the window, again. "They do know it's you. And it looks like they know it's me, as well."

"No, they don't know it's you!" said Brenda, fiercely. "I'm the one who started all of this, not you. There's no reason, no reason at all, why you should have to get nabbed for it."

"Well, it's awfully sweet of you to say so, Brenda, but I just can't let you take all of the blame for this, entirely on your own. After all, I helped you, didn't I?"

Brenda grabbed her. "Now, just you listen to me!" she cried. "I went to all that trouble of getting you out of the hospital, did I? and I didn't do it, just so you could get yourself put back in again. Where would be the sense in that? I did all of these murders, entirely on my own. Do you hear me? You had nothing whatever to do with them. You don't know anything about them at all. The only reason I'm here, now, is because we've been keeping in touch since you got out of that place. When they tell you what I've been doing, it's going to come as a complete surprise to you; it's going to come as a total shock. Do you understand me, Dorothy? Do you understand me?"

Dorothy nodded slowly. "All right, Brenda. If you absolutely insist," she said.

"Oh I do," said Brenda.

It was just at that moment, that there was a heavy knocking at the door.

"Police!" a voice called out, loudly. "Open the door, Ms. Dalton! We know you're in there!"

Releasing her hold on the other woman, Brenda said: "Go and let them in, Dorothy."

Dorothy kissed her passionately, and then went to the door.

As soon as Dorothy's back was turned, Brenda made straight for the bedroom.

Dorothy opened the door. The men came in straightaway, without waiting to be invited.

"Where's Ms. Dalton?" demanded Donaldson.

Dorothy turned round – and discovered that Brenda wasn't there any longer.

The bedroom had a window, from which one could step directly only to a fire escape. Brenda did so. She started down the stairs – and saw a policeman (the police driver) standing on the pavement below, staring up at her. She turned round and went back up the stairs, and on to the roof. She went over to the ledge.

She knew that it was only a matter of time, now…

In a strange way, she felt happy, and totally at peace. As she had said to Dorothy, she had managed to kill the worst ones of the lot: Rawsthorne, Browning, Pearson, Pattie's stepfather…

Shortly afterwards, Donaldson and Jackson made their way on to the roof (Greaves had remained behind in the flat below, to stop Dorothy from attempting to make a getaway).

Brenda place one of her feet on the ledge.

"Stop! Don't come any closer!" she cried.

It was clear what she was threatening to do. Both of the men stopped in their tracks.

She recognised Donaldson. "Hello again, Inspector," she said.

"Hello again, Brenda," he replied. "I'm very sorry we're meeting again in these particular circumstances."

"I'm sorry, too," she responded.

They exchanged glances. Her glance said: 'Are you really going to arrest me, after what we did together?' His returning glances said: 'Yes, I'm afraid so, Brenda. Sorry'.

"I suppose you know everything, of course?" she said. "Otherwise, you wouldn't be here, now."

"Yes, we know everything," Donaldson replied. "We know you and Pattie were friends at school. We know both of you were bullied by Browning and Pearson – and maybe by other girls, too, for all we know. And of course, you'd already told me about what Rawsthorne did to Pattie. Once we had found out the connection between Browning and Pearson – namely, that they were in the same class at school - it was only a matter of time before we found out everything else."

"I had hoped you wouldn't spot that particular connection," said Brenda. "That's why I left a gap of months between those two killings. Oh well – better luck next time, eh?"

Instantly, all three of them thought – but no one said – 'What next time?'

"You'll notice," Brenda went on, "that I said killings, not murders. I don't think of them as murders. When I said, just now, that I was sorry, I only meant I was sorry that I've been found out. I'm not sorry about what I did. All the people, who I killed, deserved to die. I'd do it again, if I thought that it was right." (There was no need, she thought to herself, to tell them that there already were some other people who she had been planning to kill). "And so," she concluded, "here we all are."

"Yes, here we all are," echoed Donaldson.

"Gentlemen, I've got something very important to tell you," Brenda continued. "Are both of you listening?"

"Yes, we're both listening," Donaldson replied.

"I killed Rawsthorne. And Jane Browning. And Deborah Pearson. And Pattie's stepfather. And I did it all on my own. Dorothy Little had nothing to do with any of it, absolutely nothing at all. And she doesn't know anything at all about what I've been doing. The only reason why I'm here now, is because I've been keeping in touch with her since she got out of hospital. Do you understand me?"

Again, she exchanged glances with Donaldson directly. Her glance clearly said: 'All right, Inspector, you've got me. But just be content with that. Let Dorothy go. All right?' His returning glance said, equally clearly: 'All right, Brenda'.

"Do you understand me?" Brenda repeated.

"Yes, we understand you, Brenda," replied Donaldson,

"Thank you for listening. Well, gentlemen, I don't think we've anything left to talk about." So saying, Brenda place her other foot on the ledge.

"Please, Brenda. Don't do it, for God's sake," said Donaldson. "You need help. Let us help you."

Brenda smiled ruefully.

"I think I know the sort of help Brenda smiled ruefully.

"I think I know the sort of help you mean, Inspector," she said. "You want to shut me up I that hospital, don't you? It was bad enough being a nurse in that bloody place; and now, you want to make me a patient there as well."

"But it's a much better place, now, thanks to you," said Donaldson.

"I still don't fancy going there," said Brenda. "And things might be even worse than that; I might get sent to Broadmoor." She shook her head. "Somehow, I don't think I want that to happen." She smiled her said smile again. "As they say in the movies: you'll never take me alive, copper." She waved her hand in a gesture of farewell. "Goodbye, Inspector..."

And with that, she jumped off the roof.

****

The men stared over the ledge, and looked at Brenda's shattered body, as it lay on the ground far below.

"Do you suppose Dorothy Little was in on it with her, George?" asked Jackson. "Myself, I'd take bets on it. I know Dalton said, just now, that she did it all on her own, and that Little had nothing to do with it, but I don't believe her. I think she was just covering up for Little."

"But we'll never be able to prove that," said Donaldson. "So let's just let it go, all right? And let's also let Little go."

Slowly, Jackson nodded his head in agreement. “All right, George,” he said.

Donaldson thought: Well, I’ve kept my side of our bargain, Brenda. I’ve managed to keep Dorothy out of all this.

He thought about the time when he and Brenda had made love in the back of his car – and inwardly, he started crying …

Chapter TWENTY

As Dorothy had told Brenda, both in her letter to her, and later in person – and as Inspector Donaldson had also told Brenda, on the roof of Dorothy's flat block – all of the things, that Brenda had done, had resulted in the hospital becoming a very different place now, form the place that it had used to be. Rawsthorne, of course, was long since dead. The other nurses, who had been in her clique, were long since gone; and so, too, was the man who had been the hospital's General Manager, during all of the dark days of the place's history. The hospital had been put under new management; and now, fortunately, it was a much more humane place than it had been previously.

As Inspector Donaldson had said to his colleagues, Brenda had become a local heroine, on account of all the changes that she had brought about at the hospital. Even when Brenda was publicly revealed to have been a murderess, local affection for her remained undimmed – especially when everyone learned the reasons for her crimes.

Some time later, a new ward was opened in the hospital. The occasion of the opening was marked by a special ceremony. A camera crew had been dispatched from the local television station's news programme, in order to record the even for future transmission – and possibly, for posterity as well.

The guest speaker, who had the task of opening the new ward, was none other than Dorothy Little.

"Ladies and gentlemen," she began, "I never imagined, in my wildest dreams, that I would ever be glad to set foot in this hospital again. But today, thank goodness, I'm only here as a visitor. And in any case, this place is much changed from the time when I was here as a patient. Those changes are all thanks to a certain lady. And the fact that I'm a free person today is also thanks to the same lady – her, and Inspector George Donaldson, who, I'm happy to say, is here with us today."

She exchanged smiles of greetings with the Inspector.

"So," she continued, "when I was invited here today to open this new ward, I jumped at it like a shot – especially when I found out what the ward was going to be called. I feel sure you will agree with me that, in the circumstances, there really only was one possible name for this ward. I now have great pleasure in declaring this new ward open."

So saying, Dorothy took the giant scissors that were handed to her; and to the accompaniment of applause from all of the other people who were present, she used the scissors to cut the ribbon which had been tied across the entrance of the ward.

The camera crew recorded all of it. And then the camera panned up to the sign that was heading the new ward's name:

BRENDA DALTON WARD

****

Dorothy knelt down, and placed the wreath on Brenda's grave.

At Dorothy's insistence, Brenda had been buried next to Pattie.

Dorothy was sure that it was where Brenda would have wanted to have been buried.

Getting to her feet again, Dorothy produced a sheet of paper from a pocket. It was the list, that Brenda had made, of the names and addresses of all of the girls who had bullied Pattie and Breda at school. The top two names, those of Jane Browning and Deborah Pearson, had been crossed off the list by Brenda. Dorothy contemplated the other names for a moment.

Without realising it at the time, Brenda had dropped the list on the floor of Dorothy's flat when Brenda had spent the night there. Dorothy had not noticed it until after Brenda had left, the following morning. Dorothy had been intending to return the list to Brenda, on the next occasion that she had seen her. But when Brenda had unexpectedly returned, alter that same morning, and had told Dorothy about seeing the police car that had been parked outside Brenda's flat block, all thought of the list had, naturally enough, gone out of Dorothy's mind.

"It's all right, Brenda," said Dorothy. "You may have died, but not the plans you made. I've got the list you drew up. You dropped it in my flat."

"You gave me back my freedom. You gave me back my life. And you also reformed that hospital, so that no one else would have to go through what I had to go through – or what Pattie had to go through. So the least I can do now, both for you and for Pattie, is to carry on from where the two of us left off. I'll kill all the rest of those bullies. I know who they all are, and where they all are. And I'll also kill all of those others who you mentioned. Those other nurses who were in Rawsthorne's gang. And the headmistress of your school. I'll kill every single one of them." Dorothy blew a kiss at the gravestone. "Goodbye, Brenda. God bless you. And thanks for everything."

Dorothy turned and walked away – alive and free...

THE END

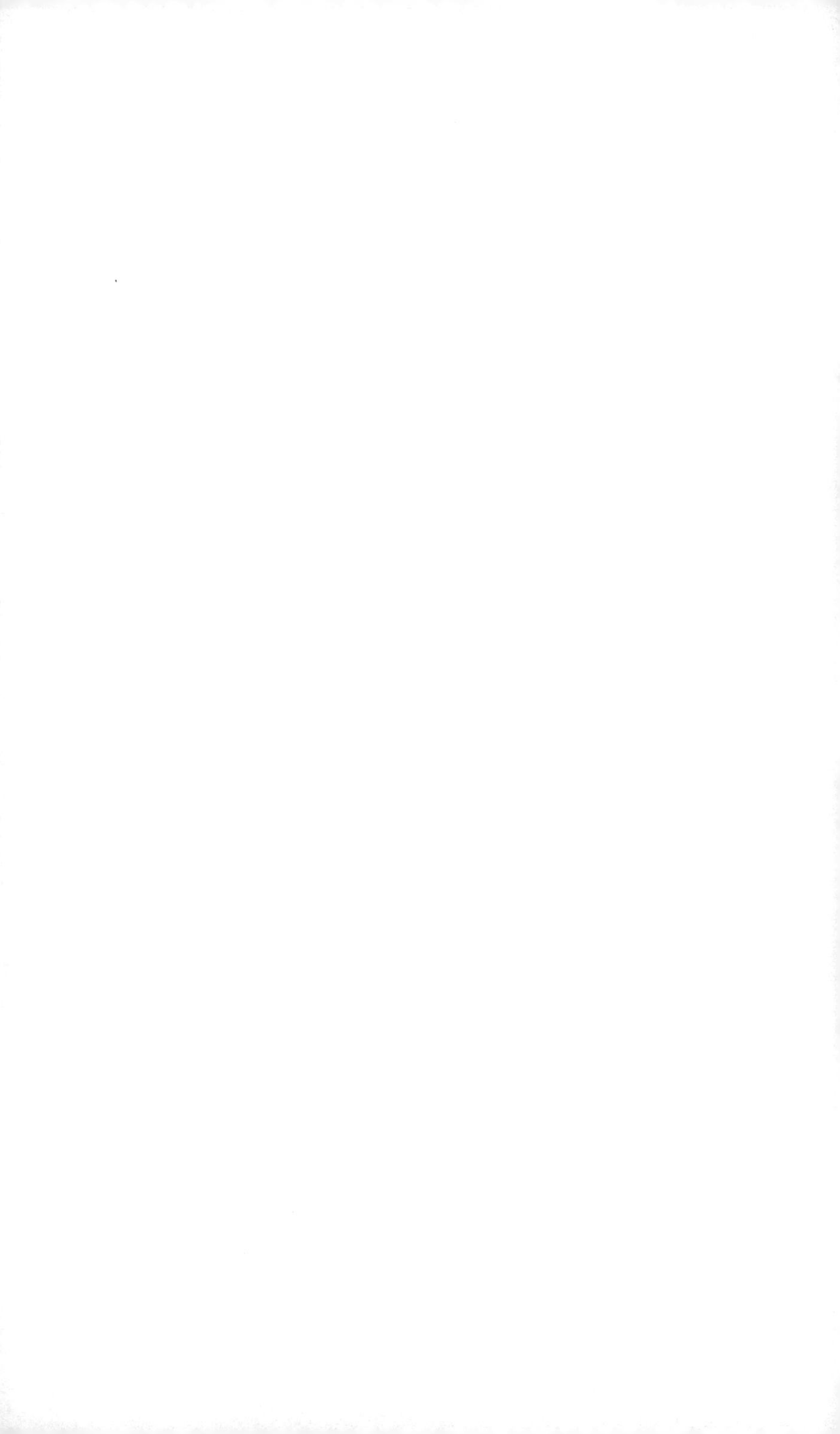

www.ingramcontent.com/pod-product-compliance
Ingram Content Group UK Ltd.
Pitfield, Milton Keynes, MK11 3LW, UK
UKHW041323190726
13851UKWH00013B/73

9 781847 478238